SpringerBriefs in Well-Being and Quality of Life Research

W0079240

SpringerBriefs in Well-Being and Quality-of-Life Research are concise summaries of cutting-edge research and practical applications across the field of well-being and quality of life research. These compact refereed monographs are under the editorial supervision of an international Advisory Board*. Volumes are 50 to 125 pages (approximately 20,000–70,000 words), with a clear focus. The series covers a range of content from professional to academic such as: snapshots of hot and/or emerging topics, in-depth case studies, and timely reports of state-of-the art analytical techniques. The scope of the series spans the entire field of Well-Being Research and Quality-of-Life Studies, with a view to significantly advance research. The character of the series is international and interdisciplinary and will include research areas such as: health, cross-cultural studies, gender, children, education, work and organizational issues, relationships, job satisfaction, religion, spirituality, ageing from the perspectives of sociology, psychology, philosophy, public health and economics in relation to Well-being and Quality-of-Life research. Volumes in the series may analyze past, present and/or future trends, as well as their determinants and consequences. Both solicited and unsolicited manuscripts are considered for publication in this series. SpringerBriefs in Well-Being and Quality-of-Life Research will be of interest to a wide range of individuals with interest in quality of life studies, including sociologists, psychologists, economists, philosophers, health researchers, as well as practitioners across the social sciences. Briefs will be published as part of Springer's eBook collection, with millions of users worldwide. In addition, Briefs will be available for individual print and electronic purchase. Briefs are characterized by fast, global electronic dissemination, standard publishing contracts, easy-to-use manuscript preparation and formatting guidelines, and expedited production schedules. We aim for publication 8–12 weeks after acceptance.

More information about this series at http://www.springer.com/series/10150

Wolfgang Glatzer

History and Politics
of Well-Being in Europe

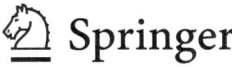 Springer

Wolfgang Glatzer
Department of Social Sciences
Goethe University
Frankfurt am Main, Germany

ISSN 2211-7644   ISSN 2211-7652 (electronic)
SpringerBriefs in Well-Being and Quality of Life Research
ISBN 978-3-030-05047-4   ISBN 978-3-030-05048-1 (eBook)
https://doi.org/10.1007/978-3-030-05048-1

Library of Congress Control Number: 2018962396

This Springer imprint is published by the registered company Springer Nature Switzerland AG
The registered company address is: Gewerbestrasse 11, 6330 Cham, Switzerland

Who is not taking into account the past three thousand years remains in his thinking in the dark and lives from the hand into the mouth
Johann Wolfgang von Goethe (1749–1832)[1]

Not to know what happened before the own birth means always to remain a child; what is the life of a human being, if it is not interwoven through history with ancient times?
Marcus Tullius Cicero (106–43 BCE)

---

[1] This proverb from Goethe is well known as well in German as in English. A number of literates have tried to translate it from German into English with different results. Above I used my own translation. The German original text is "Wer nicht von 3000 Jahren weiß sich Rechenschaft zu geben, bleibt im Inneren unerfahren, mag von Tag zu Tag leben" (Source: Pohanka 2016, p. 5). The text of Cicero above expresses the same idea about recognizing the past in Latin language: "Nescire, quid antea quam natur sis acciderit, id est semper esse puerum; quid enim est aetas hominis, nisi memoria rerum veterum com superiorum aetate contexitur?"

Dedicated to the European future of my grandchildren
Henry, Louis, Jaro, Anouk and Noëlle.

Acknowledgements

Comprehensive books like this have always many sources which exert its influence. My style of analysing was influenced preferably from two colleagues who accompanied me over long times scientifically, namely Wolfgang Zapf (25.4.1937–26.4.2018) within the research group "Micro-analytical Foundations of Society" and Karl Otto Hondrich (1.9.1937–16.1.2007) within the research team of "Comparative Charting of Social Change". Though both have passed away, their influence is still present.

That well-being has become a main topic was in the research network of ISQLS, the "International Society for Quality of Life Studies". It constitutes the context where I worked together with colleagues such as Alex Michalos, Kenneth Land, Richard Estes, Ruut Veenhoven. A special impulse to this study in Europe came from the research project on "The Pursuit of Human Well-being" organized by colleagues at Philadelphia.

Writing this book, I received much technical support from Kolja Glatzer, who produced the figures and tables. Some colleagues like Mathias Bös, Gerold Hornschu, Jürgen Kohl, Ansgar Weymann gave me advice on certain questions. The field of social indicators and quality-of-life research is a unique example of cooperation between scientific institutions and international organizations. Without the engagement of the research teams at UN, OECD, EU, EC and others, the flourishment of social indicators and quality-of-life research would not have been possible. I want to express my regards for the comprehensive knowledge transfer between social science and international institutions. Finally, I would like to say thank you to everybody who allowed me to use their data and who gave support for my work.

Contents

Chapter 1
People and Eras in European Development

Abstract Well-being of the European people in their course of history is described in many sources from the people themselves and from others, who are informed about these people. Question of well-being and quality of life in Europe concerns about 800 million people in Western and Eastern Europe, which have grown to such a high number of inhabitants in the past two centuries. Success of the European development is the reason why people now attained a life expectancy of 80 years. In the long run, the societal context of Europeans changed sustainably: "civilization" and "modernization" are the concepts which are mainly used to describe European long-term development. As it seems, the balance of progress and regress happened in favour of improving a lot of life.

Monitoring Well-Being: Human beings are inevitably exposed to highs and lows of well-being due to individual and collective events. Above the manifold individual situations, there are trends and tendencies of well-being running through bright, medium and dark episodes. The European continent has attained in the past millennium an extraordinary high level of well-being in global terms which is at the same time fragile and precarious. This is the description of the intermediate balance after three thousand years of human development on European territory. Well-being is a complex concept,[1] which is composed of positive components on the one side and of negative components on the other side, which are combined more or less with hopes and fears. It contains either people's views of their own lives or the evaluations of experts and informed people from outside.[2] In modern times, the measurement of well-being—as well as quality of life—is performed in representative surveys with

---

[1] The idea and the concept of well-being is manifold, widespread and goes historically back to ancient times. Today, the term exists in many languages, for example, in English but also in French as "bien-´e`tre" and in Spanish as "bien estar". In Germany, the terms "Wohlbefinden" and "Wohlfahrt" are closely related to well-being. Historically, they go back to "wol varn" in the medieval German language, which expresses to live happy (Glatzer 2001).

[2] In well-being, research investigations are concerned with the individual quality of life and the quality of societies. There was always some interest in the quality of life in historical societies but a new approach in modern times was to explore the attitudes and opinions of the people about their lives. The research perspective of this article is described intensively in the following books:

1
W. Glatzer, *History and Politics of Well-Being in Europe*, SpringerBriefs in Well-Being and Quality of Life Research, https://doi.org/10.1007/978-3-030-05048-1_1

elaborated questionnaires. Well-being is mainly directed towards positive concepts of well-being but it is unavoidable to include also the negative side, which develops within societies often independently from positive components.[3] Performance and contentment in Europe are high but Europeans make nevertheless a lot of complaints about their lives. The challenge for well-being policies is endless including a double task of improving well-being and alleviating misery.

Europe's people: The view of this study is concentrated on people living on the European continent in West and East. The usual demographic processes in Europe of being born and passing away are major influences of well-being. A healthy birth—5,114,128 cases in the EU in 2016[4]—is usually associated with a lot of happiness and increases the well-being of people.[5] A "happy birthday" is not only the wish for the actual birthday; moreover, it is celebrated each year through the life and contributes thus symbolically to the goal of happiness. Happiness is expressed not at least in the eyes of children. This celebration of birthdays is a historical product and a milestone in the recognition of the individual and its right for well-being.

The contrast of births is deaths which are normally associated with sadness and sorrow. There were in 2016 a number of 5,129,982 people passing away in Europe, and consequently, this reduced well-being day by day. The idea of "quality of life" did not end with the death of human beings; moreover, it was expanded by the concept of "quality of dying and death" (Curtis et al. 2012). A "good death" is part of the quality of life.

In the last centuries, the number of births went most often above the number of deaths and thus the EU population grew. The population of Europe in ancient times was much smaller than today and shifted around 25 million (Fig. 1.1). People in Europe—397 in Western Europe and 407 in Eastern Europe—count in 2000 nearly 804 million together, and the expectation is sometimes that 1000 million will be attained at the end of the ongoing century. What problems this will generate for the well-being of European people is a challenging question.

The long-term development of the European population Before the Current Era (abbreviated BCE)[6] was characterized by stagnation. The first millennium CE was accompanied by a low population growth, but later happened in the second millennium CE an increase during medieval time. Finally, Europe's demography became

---

Lanc et al. (2012), Glatzer et al. (2015), Estes and Sirgy (2017). A pre-study of this work is available in G atzer and Kohl (2017).

[3]In each language, dozens of words are available to make distinctions between various positive states of well-being and also between many different negative states of well-being. As a consequence, we find 35 items for well-being in the European survey of 2012.

[4]https://www.ined.fr/en/everything_about_population/data/europe-developed-countries/population-births-deaths/.

[5]In special cases a positive event like a birth may be evaluated negative and a negative event like a death can be evaluated positive but these are exceptional cases

[6]Current Era and Common Era (CE in both cases) is a religious neutral expression for AD (After Domini), which depends on the Gregorian calendar. Before the Current Era is equivalent to Before the Common Era (BCE) and BC (Before Christ).

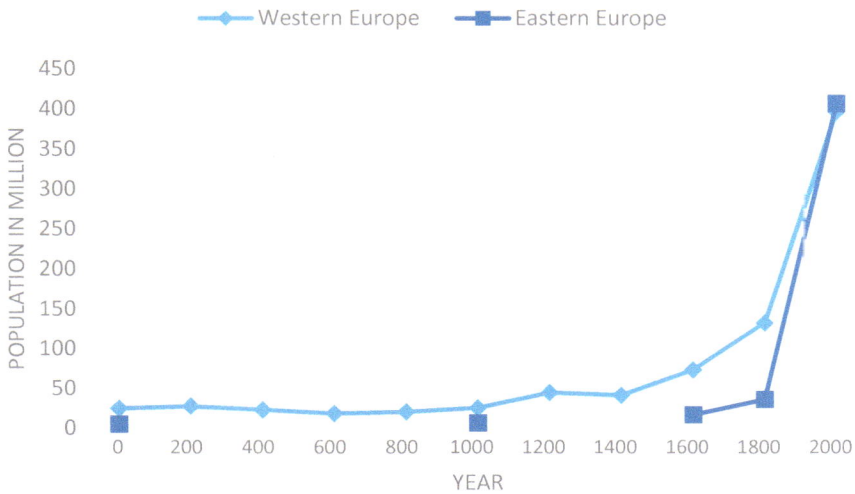

Fig. 1.1 Population development in Western and Eastern Europe in the past millennia from 0 to 2000. *Sources* Own diagram according to data of Maddison (2001), p. 32, 232 (0–1600); Van Zanden et al. (2014), p. 42 (1800–2000) (data for Eastern Europe are partly not available; the data for 1800 are substituted by 1820)

mobile and an explosion of population numbers emerged in modern times first in Western and then in Eastern Europe (Fig. 1.1).

The number of Europeans grew mainly during the demographic transition close to the middle of the eighteenth century (Flora 1987). During the past millennium, the population raised 25-fold from close to 30 million (Maddison 2001, p. 232) up to 784 million (Van Zanden et al. 2014, p. 42). In the same time—accompanying the population growth—life expectancy of European people doubled in the average. All countries in Western Europe were affected in a similar way. In the course of this population growth, Western Europe went always ahead of Eastern Europe but in recent times the number of Eastern Europe people attained the population of number Western Europe. The number of people in Europe grew, the length of life for the individuals increased at the same time, and less people—among the adults and the children—passed away. This seems to be basic progress for people's well-being in Europe (Fig. 1.2).

The demographic development reflects the decrease of destroying factors for well-being. A reduction of mortality especially of infant mortality diminished the sorrows caused by higher number of deaths in earlier times. With some delay to the reduction of mortality followed a decrease of birth rates, contributing at the end to a diminished population growth. This was called the demographic wave which led to a new balance of the demographic development between births and deaths. All European countries followed this demographic process. It was an increase of well-being that less people died and more people lived longer, but there came also the critical question if the

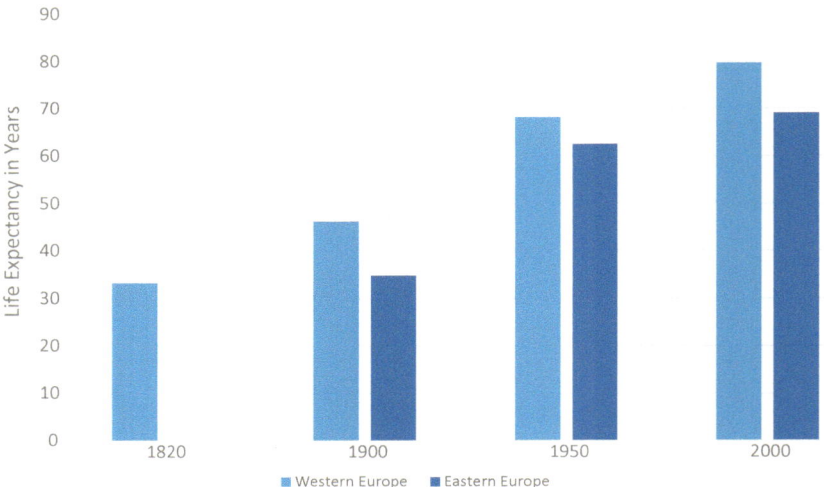

Fig. 1.2 Life expectancy at birth for Western and Eastern Europeans from 1820 to 2000. *Source* Own diagram with data from Van Zanden et al. (2014), p. 108

prolongation of life, which is basically perceived as positive, was really an increase of a good life.

European's Eras: The time span of this investigation goes roughly spoken through 3000 years,[7] 1000 years before and 2000 years after the Common Era (Black 2005). A few exceptions are going beyond this time window. The most famous old culture mentioned sometimes as an origin of Europe is the Minoan civilization which flourished on the island of Crete in a time between 2600 and 1200 CE. The somewhat younger cultural highlight was the Mycenaean civilization on the mainland of Greece from 1600 to 1100. In both cases, a high performance with respect to architecture and arts is documented but we have only little knowledge how far "well-being" was a concern in these ancient cultures.

Within and around the millennium before the Common Era—and about five hundred years after—was more or less characterized in Europe by five ancient civilizations: the Celts, the Greeks, the Romans and the Germanic tribes in the Western Europe, and the Slavs in the Eastern Europe. As far as we know, all together had developed different styles of living combined with specific traits of well-being. Through several hundred years, these civilizations dominated in large parts of Europe and above in North Africa and Near East.

A relative turbulent era for Europe began at the end of the Roman Empire, which was conquered finally by Germanic tribes. A number of Germanic tribes participated in European migration movements, which endured some hundred years. Germanic

---

[7]The time window of 3000 years was introduced by Johann Wolfgang Goethe as it is shown in his proverb on the first page of this book, but it makes a lot of sense due to the traditional knowledge which we have.

tribes came from the North and migrated partly until North Africa, building every-where new territorial areas. It is not well known what push and pull factors were motivating tribes and peoples to participate in the long-distance migrations. The question is sometimes asked, if the unrest, which is a basic motivation of the multi-fold migration movements, was caused by dissatisfaction due to the deterioration of living conditions and deficits of well-being.

After three hundred years of migration trouble emerged a new pattern of territo-ries and kingdoms in Europe. It was the Merovingian dynasty, which prepared the unification of broad territories of Central Europe. Finally, the Franconian Empire of Charlemagne constituted a stable and mighty empire for about 40 years. Most charac-terizing for the Franconian Empire are medieval prosperity and cultural renaissance.

The dissolution of the Franconian Empire beginning with the division among the sons of Charlemagne led to a multi-fragmented Europe landscape. It is said that around 1000 CE, the picture of the distribution of European countries emerged similar to the state of today (Black 2005).

Europeans human development is sometimes characterized in comprehensive terms, in this case "civilization" and "modernization" are the preferably used con-cepts. The usual lexical definition of "Western civilization" happens as follows.

> "**Western civilization** traces its roots back to Western Europe and the Western Mediterranean. It is linked to the Roman Empire and with Medieval Western Christendom which emerged from the Middle Ages to experience such trans-formative episodes as the Renaissance, the Reformation, the Enlightenment, the Industrial Revolution, scientific revolution, and the development of liberal democracy. The civilizations of Classical Greece, Ancient Rome, and Ancient Israel[1] are considered seminal periods in Western history; a few cultural con-tributions also emerged from the pagan peoples of pre-Christian Europe, such as the Celts and Germans. Christianity and Roman Catholicism has played a prominent role in the shaping of Western civilization, which throughout most of its history, has been nearly equivalent to Christian culture."[8]

The concept of civilization is in dispute because it is often related to a certain superiority of Europe (Ferguson 2011). It is still in broad use—not at least in everyday language—but in the course of time it was substituted primarily in the social sciences by the concept of modernization.[9] Modernization approaches are comprehensive

---

[8]https://en.wikipedia.org/wiki/History_of_Western_civilization. There exists a comprehensive meaning of "civilization", as it is expressed in the citation from Wikipedia above. This under-standing of civilization belongs surely to the most widespread definitions.

[9]The socio-economic development of Europe and other modern countries is preferably described as "modernization" (Mau and Verwiebe 2009), and the recent era is designed as "modernity" (Hall et al. 1996) and the newest era is designed as "postmodern". Historical ethnologists speak of the modernization of Europe as a "singular" process that traces its roots to the beginning of the past millennium.

concepts for long-term societal development which accept that alternative ways of modernization exist. They can be summarized as follows:

"**Modernization** … designs a complex of interrelated structural, cultural and individual changes, which began in the early Modern Time and is prolonged and increased in the twentieth century. It includes processes like industrialization, rationalization and secularization, democratization and emancipation, individualization and pluralization of life styles, mass consumption and growth, urbanization and increase of social mobility. Such processes of modernization influence in Western societies still the direction of societal development from plain rural to complex and differentiated industrial societies" (Degele 2014, p. 326).

Each of the concepts mentioned in these descriptions is of broad meaning, captures many developmental theories and sees a positive outcome for human development. They are opposed to Marxist theory, which defines history as class struggle moved forward by the productive forces and their relationships to production. The consequence of Marxist theory is in the end a tendency towards impoverishment. On the other side, sociologists point out that modernization was an universal, multidimensional process of social change in Europe characterized by the Industrial Revolution in England (1760–1830) and the Political Revolution in France (1789–1794) (Bendix 1969). These were indeed most important social-historical events and processes, which spread in the course of time in Europe and above contributing to the well-being of populations. There were always some pioneer societies taking the lead and some latecomer societies trailing behind. Altogether is concluded that modernization, following after millennia of stagnation, had overwhelmingly positive effects on people's welfare (Zapf 1979). The mixture of improvement and deterioration in the historical processes is in the final balance regarded as overwhelmingly positive despite many losses.

Well-being in Europe surely missed to attain an optimal level of quality of life for all the people; it went moreover through valleys and over hills and diminished in the end the threats for the well-being of large numbers of people.

References

Bendix, R. (1969). Modernisierung in internationaler Perspektive. In W. Zapf (Ed.), *Theorien des sozialen Wandels* (pp. 505–512). Kiepenheuer & Witsch, Köln.
Black, J. (2005). *Dumont Atlas of World History*. London: Dorling Kindersley.
Curtis, J. R., Patrick, D. L., Engelberg, R. A., Norris, K., Asp, C., & Byock, I. (2012). A measure of the quality of dying and death. *PUbMedResult, 43*(2), 195–204.
Estes, R., & Sirgy, J. (2017). *The pursuit of human well-being*. Switzerland: Springer International Publishing.

Degele, N. (2014). Modernisierung. In G. Endruweit, G. Trommsdorf, N. Burzan (Hg.), Wörterbuch der Soziologie. (3 ed., pp. 326–329), Stuttgart: Lucius & Lucius (UTB).

Ferguson, N. (2011). *Civilization: The West and the Rest*. London: Penguin Group.

Flora, P. (1987). *State, Economy and Society in Western Europe. Vol. II, The Growth of Industrial Societies and Capitalist Economies*. Campus Verlag, Frankfurt

Glatzer, W. (2001). Wohlfahrt in der Wohlfahrtsgesellschaft. In H. Hill (Ed.), *Modernisierung—Prozess oder Entwicklungsstrategie?* Frankfurt, New York: Campus.

Glatzer, W., Camfield, L., Moller, V., & Rojas, M. (Eds.). (2015). *Global handbook of quality of life*. Dordrecht: Springer.

Glatzer, W., Kohl, J. (2017). The history of well-being in Europe. In R. Estes, J. Sirgy (Eds.), *The Pursuit of Human Well-Being*. Switzerland: Springer.

Hall, S., Held, D., Hubert, D., & Thompson, K. (1996). *Modernity. An Introduction to Modern Societies*. Massachusetts: Blackwell Publisher.

Land, K.C., Michalos, A.C., Sirgy, M.J. (2012). *Handbook of Social Indicators and Quality of Life Research*. Dordrecht Heidelberg, London, New York: Springer

Maddison, A. (2001). *The world economy. A millennial perspective*. Paris: OECD.

Mau, S., & Verwiebe, R. (2009). *Die Sozialstruktur Europas*. Konstanz: UVK.

Van Zanden, J., et al. (Eds.). (2014). *How was life? Global well-being since 1820*. Paris: OECD Publishing.

Zapf, W. (1979). Modernization and welfare development: The case of Germany. *Social Science Information, 18*(2), 219–246.

Chapter 2
Geographical Benefits for the European Continent

Abstract Geographic position and the shape of the European continent: Europe is a part of the double-continent Eurasia (Europe and Asia), but for a long time, it has been most often recognized as a continent of its own. Compared with other continents, Europe's territory was in the long run better protected from "natural" disasters. Europe is situated in a way which offers in large parts of natural advantages with respect to climate and weather. Of special importance is Europe's warming up by the Gulf Stream, which is designed as the "natural heating system". In most parts, the European continent offers a favourable environment for the well-being of its people but climate change has become a threat to the future of the continent.

From geological and geographic views, Europe is a part of the double-continent Eurasia (Europe and Asia) but since a long time, it has been most often recognized as a continent of its own (Dumont and Verluise 2016). Europe's natural borders are roughly described: the Atlantic Ocean in the West, the Arctic Ocean in the North, the Ural Mountains in the East and the Mediterranean Sea in the South. Europeans are at most positions close to the sea, and they used this in their history as starting points for exploring and conquering the world.

According to Europe's proximity to the big oceans, it shows four different climate zones, namely continental climate (in the East of Central Europe), maritime climate (in the West of Central Europe), subtropical zone (in the South of Europe) and polar zone (in the North of Europe). Most territories of Europe are classified as temperate because they expose people to amenable climate conditions with moderate changes between summer and winter. The problem lays in the emergence of natural risks insofar "humanity has become more and more vulnerable to long—and short-term climate change" (Fagan 2004, p. xvii).

Geographers have argued that geographic conditions are an important source for "the wealth and poverty of nations" (Landes 1999). In the case of Europe, the amenable climate is a great benefit of the monumental "Gulf Stream", which comes from the Middle American Atlantic coast and goes far into the North, creating on its way a decent climate for large areas of Europe (Fig. 2.1).

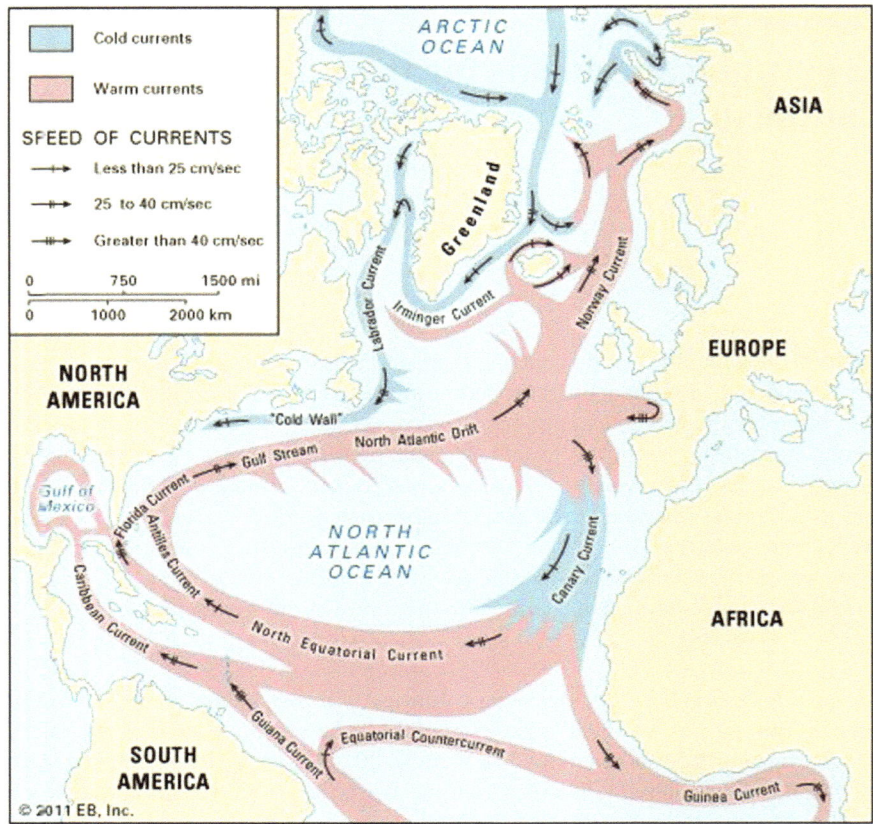

Fig. 2.1 Gulf Stream: Europe's natural heating system. *Source* https://www.britannica.com/science/climate-meteorology/The-Gulf-Stream

This called a "natural heating system", which brings substantial advantages for the well-being of the European population. In the eyes of the expert, the geographic situation of Europe is evaluated in terms of well-being a "privileged European climate" and a "favourable environment" (Landes 1999, pp. 18, 20).

All in all, Europe is an exceptional continent with some preconditions for a positive well-being. It does not have the amount of natural threats which lead other continents again and again to large catastrophes. Tsunamis, earthquakes, tornados, hurricanes, volcanoes eruptions and bush fires are sometimes present but not as many as in elsewhere continents. There are in Europe relatively few hot zones and ice areas. But surprises are never excluded as the hot century summer of 2018.

With respect to its geographic situation and its natural environment, Europe is, when compared to other continents, in a privileged position. But the existing burden is not equally distributed among Europeans and a variety of geographic conditions between the warm South and the cold North in Europe have influenced the socio-economic development in the past. Lately, the apprehension grows that the ongoing climate change associated with an increase of the water levels and an increase of temperature is a severe threat to the well-being and could lead in the long run to a downfall of significant parts of Europe (European Environment Agency Report 2012). The disputes about these risks are intensively carried through in recent years especially with the engagement of natural and social sciences. There are severe strains in various countries to protect from the dangers to attain future well-being.

According to socio-geographic experts, the geological and geographic context of Europeans' well-being is a donation of nature but its future development lies in the hands of the peoples and its climate policies.

References

Dumont, G., & Verluise, P. (2016). *The geopolitics of Europe—From the Atlantic to the Urals*. Kindle Edition.
European Environment Agency. (2012). *Climate change, impacts and vulnerability in Europe 2012*. An Indicator-based Report, No. 12/2012.
Fagan, B. (2004). *The long Summer: How climate changed civilization*. Basic Books.
Landes, D. S. (1999). *The wealth and poverty of nations*. New York: Norton.

Chapter 3
The Awareness of Europeans in Ancient Times

Abstract In its past, Europe and Europeans were perceived as very different from today. Early European continent was an unknown territory in the North of the Mediterranean Sea, and its population was from the view of Greek's high culture called "barbarians". Europe was explored step by step, beginning with the voyages of Pytheas of Massilia to the North of Europe. Barbarians surrounding the Greek people were perceived as people of inferior culture, bad habits, uncivilized, primitive and cruel. Though Europe has made civilizational steps forward to higher cultural levels the threat though all kind of new barbarians have remained all the time a challenge for the continent and the world.

Europe's early cartographic representation is a wide territory in the North of the Mediterranean Sea (see Fig. 3.1). The naming of Europe is not obvious. "Europe" was in antique Greek mythology a mistress of the mighty god Zeus and sometimes in the literature it is told that her name was lent to the continent Europe.[1]

In the early awareness of Europe, it was an unexplored and hidden territory whose people were defined as "barbarians", which is the ancient Greek perception of the inferior civilizations of the non-Greeks. "Barbarism" can be regarded as an ancient contrast term for "well-being". The well-being history of Europe began with the old-fashioned story of the high civilization of the Greeks in contrast to the inferior cultures of the Barbarians around them. The topic of well-being was already significant among the famous Greek philosophers and the starting point for the West European civilization.

An imagination of "Europe" and its well-being developed slowly during the past millenniums. Already in the works of the Greek historian Herodot (484–424 BCE), the territories in the North of Greece were designed as "Europe". Together with "Asia" and "Libya", there were three continents at this time, which were situated around the Mediterranean Sea. Greek city states constituted the centre of this small world. In writings of Herodot, Europe has been designated a "continent", though its contours were not well known (Mitchell 2007). It was the Greek explorer Pytheas of Massilia (380–310 BCE) who undertook around 330 BCE exploring shipping tours

---

[1] en.wikipedia.org/wiki/Europe tells this story, which varies sometimes.

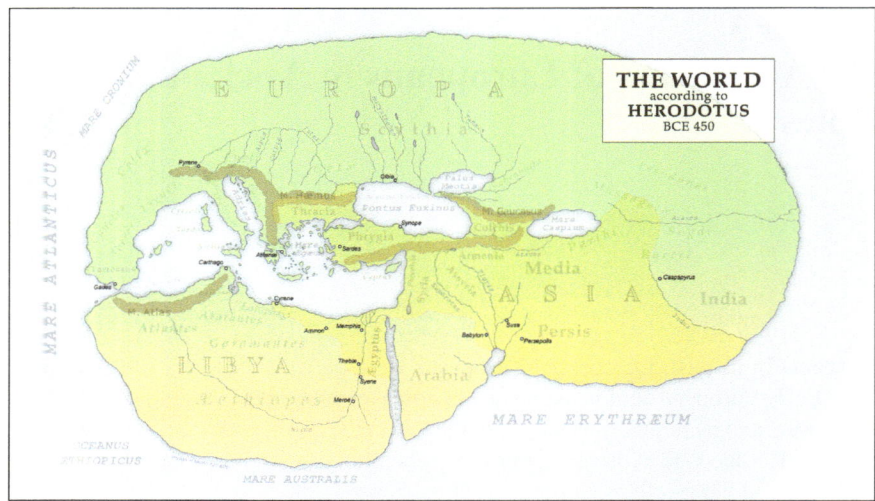

Fig. 3.1 Herodotus World Map—Greek civilization at the Mediterranean Sea (Centre Athens) surrounded by barbarian peoples. *Source* http://www.meer.org/ebook/herodotus-world-map-1a.jpg

into the hidden North. He was presumably the first explorer[2] who created a rough map of the non-discovered land in the North-West of Europe. He was also speaking of the foreign European people in the North-West as "barbarians" (Tozer 1897).

"Barbarians" were perceived as a prototype of "negative well-being" and preferably described as cruel, terrible, evil, uncivilized, violent and primitive. If this was the truth or not was secondary compared with functions and consequences with respect to the people who were labelled as barbarians. The barbarians were one of the first broadly used negative stereotypes for people in ancient times who were perceived as missing culture and well-being.

From the view of well-being, the question was sometimes asked "how barbaric were the barbarians?" Surely barbarian stereotypes were founded with a certain degree of prejudice. But no doubt that barbarian behaviour existed as a problematic part of mankind. The expectation was never realized that barbarian behaviour did fully disappear.

As it looks today, there were different types and degrees of civilizations in Europe which developed further. Also, plain civilizations upgraded in the course of time. A chain of civilizational steps led in the long run to what is later called the "European or Western civilization".

---

[2]It is assumed up and on that there were explorers of Europe some time before Pytheas but obviously they did not sail far enough into the North. His travel reports were criticized from historians of the time, but according to modern reconstruction of his journeys he seems to be right.

References

Mitchell, L. (2007). *Panhellenism and the Barbarian in Archaic and Classical Greece*.
Tozer, H. F. (1897). *A history of ancient geography*. Cambridge: University Press.

Chapter 4
Heritage of Early European Peoples: Celts, Greeks, Romans, Germanics and Slavs

Abstract Large civilizations were characterizing the European continent in the millennia before and after the year 0. They were partly independent, partly in conflict and partly in cooperation. They had their high times at different points of history, and they have prepared valuable goods and transferred them into modern times. From the Greeks stem theatre, democracy, philosophy and the Olympic Games, the Celts have built the first toll-free long-distance roads, the Romans have organized the Pax Romana, which was a long unique peacetime, Germanic tribes supported in Northern Europe sustainable attitudes towards woods and forest. Not at least the Slavs have shown how to overcome in a more difficult region of Europe and to grow to the biggest European language group.

Europe is a continent, where various large populations have settled during the past three millenniums. Europe's long ways into the civilized world emerged on the background of the early peoples of Greeks, Romans, Celts, Germanics and Slavs. The people at the beginning of this time have created a heritage for our modern quality of life which is virulent up today. Most prominent is this in the characterization of the Greek high culture as the "birthplace of Western civilization". There were five big populations on European territories: Celts, Greeks, Romans, Germanics and Slavs, and all were speaking different Indo-European Languages.[1] It was not seldom that they fought battles against one another and at some time, they organized cooperation. They were reaching their height in terms of culture and power at different points of time. Do they influence the quality of life of today? The answer of the historical research of today is for Greece without doubt: "Ancient Greece was the birthplace of advances in government, art, philosophy, science, and architecture—all of which

---

[1] They developed their own ways of life and constituted different forms of associations: in respect to the large populations of the last 3000 year in Europe, there is a rich and relatively well-documented history for Greeks and Romans in writings but for Celts and Germanics without writings. In the literature, it is usual to regard the heritage of Greeks and Romans but not the one of Celts and Germanic culture and the Slav people are recognized at least.

W. Glatzer, *History and Politics of Well-Being in Europe*, SpringerBriefs in Well-Being and Quality of Life Research, https://doi.org/10.1007/978-3-030-05048-1_4

continue to influence the world today" (Kitto 1991, p. 7). Did the other tribes influence our modern quality of life? There are a number of hints in the historical literature that this is true. The ancient populations are described according to their timelines as follows:

The **Celtic** culture ranging roughly from 1400 BCE to 4 CE which is from the first Celtic cultures at the upper Danube in Central Europe until the funeral of Herod II, which marked an endpoint of Celtic power[a] (Schaper 2011).

The **Greek** civilization, mainly city states, executed broad influence from the Archaic Period around 800 BCE until the end of the Hellenistic period at 146 BCE.[b] They were beaten by the Romans (Kitto 1991).

The **Roman** Empire ranges from 45 BCE, when Caesar became the first dictator, constituted the most powerful Empire around the Mediterranean Sea and existed until 476 CE, when the last emperor of West Rome was disposed by the Gothic King Odoacer[c] (Woolf 2012).

Germanic tribes were settling and migrating in Europe from 200 BCE up to the end of the fifth century CE. The "Limes" constituted the border between the Roman Empire and Germanic tribes which was from Germanic warriors under Arminius the Cheruscian destroyed in the battle in the Teutoburger Woods (Schaper 2008).

Slavs were the biggest ethnolinguistic group in Europe which concentrated themselves from 1500 BCE onwards on wide territories of Eastern Europe. They established their settlements and founded afterwards states which had to resist in the first line the Hun occupation form East Asia. Today they exist in states speaking Slavic languages, for example, Russia, Serbia, Montenegro joined by Poland, Croatia, Slovenia and Slovakia (Dvornik 1992).

[a]Celts were people who spoke Celtic languages and were similar in cultural respect. Their homeland is seen in the Hallstatt culture in Austria. They expanded by transcultural diffusion and migration to the British Iles, France and Gaul, Bohemia and Poland, much of Central Europe, the Iberian Peninsula and the North of Italy, the Gaels and the Celtic Britons Angles
[b]Greece at this time was situated in the South-East of Europe and embraced also certain areas of Turkey, the Mediterranean Sea Coast, Italy, Sicily, North Africa and West France. At its height, Greece was constituted of numerous city states
[c]The Imperial Roman period ranges over a time span of nearly 500 years. At the height of the Imperial period, the Roman Empire had conquered most of the known world—North Africa (Morroco, Egypt), Gaul, Spain, parts of Germany, Britain, Central Europe and parts of Western Asia

---

It is an important sign for a leading quality of life that others were following the Greek example immediately and in the long run-up to the modern world of today. Of course it should be not forgotten that seen from today, there is also massive criticism. For example, Greek democracy excluded women from politics and slavery was a regular concomitant of society. Nevertheless, this is not denying the basic significance of the Greek model.

4.1   Overview 1: Heritages of Early European Tribes: Celts, Greeks, Romans, Germanics

Celts

- **Document I: Celt Roads**

"The Celts had created great road networks through Europe for trade and expansion, long before the Romans. …The Celts expanded their trading network throughout Europe and traded in luxury goods. At this time the Celts created the famous Tin Road which began in Massalia and spread to Britain and the Amber Road through the Moravian Gate into modern day Danzig. …Yet this roadbuilding skill was not only used for long distance trade." (Robb 2014)

Greeks

- **Document II: The Greek Model**

"About 2500 years ago, the Greeks created a way of life that other people admired and copied. …The Ancient Greeks tried out democracy, started the Olympic Games and left new ideas in science, art and philosophy (thinking about life)." Especially Greek theatre received high recognition. "Thus the work of such great playwrights as Sophokles and Aristophanes formed the foundation upon which all modern theatre is based". "Greeks took their way of life to many places."
www.bbc.co.k/schools/primaryhistory/ancient-greeks/greek_world/ and www.ancient.eu/Greek_Theatre/

Romans

- **Document III: The Pax Romana**

"The Pax Romana (Roman Peace) was a period of relative peace and stability across the Roman Empire which lasted for over 200 years." It is emphasized "This was a time of peace and prosperity in the Roman Empire". Additional it is explained "The stability generated under Augustus brought a sense of satisfaction." Overall the description is "Rome`s citizen were relative secure and the government generally maintained law, order, and stability." (Goldsworthy 2014)

Germanics

- **Document IV: Germanic Wood Conservation**

"A land whose surface was probably covered by forest impressed Roman observers. …Permanent towns and villages were a rarity in Free Germania. Settlements would be abandoned after a period of time and biological succession set in. This enabled a return of vegetation to something resembling its natural state."

Before: "Roman colonization saw the first drastic impact on the forest communities of Central Europe. It left forest free areas, that did not recover from grazing."
https://en.wikipedia.org/wiki/History_of_the_forest_in_Central_Europe

It is difficult to overview the multiple heritages which were resulting from the Roman Empire for modern quality of life. There are a lot of heritages from the Roman Empire, which were not only creations by their culture but also transfers of components from predecessors like the ancient Greece peoples. Among them are famous buildings like the Roman roads and viaducts installed to secure water supply or the Roman juridical system which is at present still a model. Most attention is given to a time of peace and prosperity which is called the "Pax Romana" or "Roman Peace" which endured about 200 hundred years.

There is no doubt that components of quality of life have accumulated.

It is a long time from 27 BCE to 180 CE where the available descriptions tell that "peace, prosperity, security and satisfaction" were existing for the 70 million inhabitants of the Roman Empire. Such a long time of relative peaceful social development never happened before and after and is therefore a model for well-being in modern Europe. It receives attention that this was not the case for everybody as "the quality of life in the Roman Empire depended on the place people took in society".

The Romans were consequently blocked from an expansion into Central Europe. The military leader Varus lost with three Roman legions the famous battle in the "Teutoburg Forest" against the Germanic allied troop under Arminius (9 CE). One explanation for the Germanic success is that the Germanic tribes were better capable to arrange themselves with the conditions of the woods.

The Germanic tribes had developed another behaviour towards woods and forests than the Romans. Whereas the Romans exploited the woods as far as possible, for the Germanic tribes, the re-naturalization was a usual behaviour. But the history of the European forests is complex though the footsteps of the past are still recognizable. We find nowadays a very high wood ratio in the North of Europe where Romans never arrived, for example, in Finland and Sweden. Below the Limes, which was the border between Romans and Germanics in Central and Western Europe, the forests are often scarce and small or middle wood ratios exist after recreation in many centuries.[2]

With respect to the ancient Slavic tribes, their relevance and influence for modern quality of life seem to be concentrated in Eastern Europe where they dominated continually. Slavs were in comparison with other populations, the largest group in Europe, and they kept their place continually and were relatively isolated from West European history. Remarkable to mention that their well-being suffered first in Europe under the attacks of the Huns coming from East Asian territories to conquer wide areas of Europe.

There are contributions to our modern quality of life since the Antique in Europe. They were developed in ancient times and modified through the centuries and adapted to modern societies in recent times.

References

Dvornik, F. (1992). *The Slavs in European history and civilization*. Rutgers University Press.
Goldsworthy, A. (2014). *Pax Romana—War, peace and conquest in the Roman World*. Yale University Press.
Kitto, H. (1991). *The Greeks*. Penguin History.

---

[2]Especially German identity is often defined in a symbolic connection with woods and their link to nature. The concept of "sustainability" is obviously stemming from principles of wood managing in Germany. Sustainability is derived from wood managing: do not cut more wood than it grows again.

Robb, G. (2014). *The ancient paths—Discovering the lost map of Celtic Europe*. London: Macmillan.

Schaper, M. (2008). *Die Germanen: Wie sie lebten, woran sie glaubten, weshalb sie kämpften: Der Aufstiege einer rätselhaften Völkerschar*. GEO Epoche 34/08.

Schaper, M. (2011). *Die Kelten – Fürsten, Krieger und Druiden*. GEO Epoche 47.

Woolf, G. (2012). *Rome—An empires story*. Oxford: Oxford University Press.

Chapter 5
Wars and the Destruction of Well-Being

Abstract In the past 2000 years, wars have been the main factors deteriorating and destroying well-being. Nevertheless, wars have been affecting Europeans history again and again. Wars of short and long duration (up to hundred years) with thousands and millions of war deaths were part of European history. Wars between European nations played a major role, but also wars inside of nations and wars with "enemies" abroad happened again and again. In many cases, influential groups gave war goals priority to peace goals and well-being goals. It must be seen as a victory for the peaceful forces that after the founding of the European Union the number of wars decreased. Death is in general detracting well-being. Historically, in addition to the deterioration caused by wars, well-being in Europe was diminished by plagues and epidemics and not at least by the prosecution of "witchcrafts". Also in modern time, continuing causes of death are going on, like traffic deaths and suicides.

The unavoidability of death is a natural law which sets principal limits for human beings to attain a very high satisfaction with life. Always people are passing away and this is usually accompanied by grief and sorrow and thus in a loss of well-being. In the face of death, all human beings are equal, yet it makes a significant difference how people come to death: people often accept death more easy as a natural event and claim about man-made fatalities by aggression, accidents, conflicts and wars. Wars were without doubt a significant source of man-made fatalities and brutality.[1] That they sometimes increase the well-being of parts of people belongs to the paradoxical surprises of wars (Bös and Rosenbrock 2015, p. 92). It is not easy to find long periods without any wars on Europe's territory during the past millenniums. The famous historic exception is the 200 years of prevailing peace during the Pax Romana. On the other side, there are long lists of some hundred wars and different types of conflict in Europe, in detail wars between European states, civil wars within European states, wars between a European state and a non-European state that took place within Europe and global conflicts in which Europe was the area of war. More

---

[1] It is difficult to express in scientific writings the brutality and cruelty of wars and their negative consequences for the well-being of people. It is especially a capability of artisans to hint to the cruelty of wars as Picasso did it (Müller 2018). "Guernica" is perhaps his most influential picture.

© The Author(s), under exclusive licence to Springer Nature Switzerland AG 2019   23
W. Glatzer, *History and Politics of Well-Being in Europe*, SpringerBriefs in Well-Being and Quality of Life Research, https://doi.org/10.1007/978-3-030-05048-1_5

thar 800 conflicts and wars were counted in the European list which ranges from the first to the twenty-first[2] century. This implies that states and peoples had strongest difficulties to live in peace with another. The wars were very different with respect to their duration and the number of fatalities which resulted from the wars.[3] Six wars in Europe's last two millenniums, which increased steadily their technology of weapons, caused according to expert estimations above one million fatalities. Especially the two World Wars, which are in the responsibility of Germany, brought millions of deaths and sadness and sorrow about Europe.

5.1 Overview 2: Wars in Europe with One Million Fatalities and More

One Hundred Years' War (1337–1453): Historians collected a series of battles between the kingdoms of England and France about the succession of the French throne to the longest war of mankind. France lost half its population during the Hundred Years' War. Normandy lost three-quarters of its population, and Paris two-thirds. The population of England was reduced by 20–33% due to plague in the same period.

(Fatalities: 0.5–3.0 million)

Thirty Years' War (1618–1648): A brutal religious war in Central Europe with many conflict lines especially between Catholic and Protestant states involving all great powers in Europe. After long-term suffering of broad populations, the war was finished with the Peace of Westphalia, which is a height in difficult peace-making.

(Fatalities: 3.0–11.5 million)

The Seven Years' War (1756–1763): This war was global and the great powers from five countries were involved with the kingdoms of England and France as central opponents. It was a key moment in Prussia's rise to greatness. Though Prussia's lands and population were devastated, Frederick's extensive agrarian reforms and encouragement of immigration solved these problems.

(Fatalities: 0.9–1.4 million)

Napoleonic Wars (1803–1815): A number of separated conflicts performed from the French empire led by Napoleon against various European coalitions. Spain as well as Germany and Russia were the places of big battles. The fights about the military dominance in Europe went from victories of Napoleon to its defeat at Waterloo.

(Fatalities: 3.5–6.0 million)

(continued)

---

[2]https://en.wikipedia.org/wiki/List_of_conflicts_in_Europe.

[3]Beside the long-term wars there were long-during regional conflicts which were disturbing peace in Western Europe for example North Ireland, the Basque Country, South Tyrol, and various short-term revolts in Eastern Europe as in the German Democratic Republic 1953, in Hungary 1956, in Prague 1969. They cannot be explained without regarding the dissatisfaction of the populations.

(continued)

World War I (1914–1918): This global war, originating in Europe, was the first one of worldwide warfare which killed people not only in Europe but around the world. The destruction of well-being experienced a new increase by technical advanced weapons especially with the use of chemical weapons against international agreements.
(Fatalities: 20 million)
World War II (1939–1945): This was the most widespread war in history which included all great nations. Beginning 1 September 1939 with the German attack on Poland it grew to a worldwide fight between Axis powers and Allied forces. It was finished with the defeat of Germany after having caused a death rate higher as never before.
(Fatalities: 40–85 million)

Wars exercise their negative influence on well-being not only by killing people during the fights, but they bring often anxiety and fears over the countries, leave wounded people after the battles, destroy much of the infrastructure, which people need. The damages are often not reconstructed before the next war comes, and the people have to carry war-related financial burden. Well-being is usually destructed before and after wars and beside the wars and as well conflicts were many additional destroyers as described below.

Plagues and epidemics have killed millions of people in medieval times. Sometimes in severe pandemics, the death toll was more than half of the European population. There were different styles of spread as occasional, sporadic, endemic and pandemic. The sources of the infection diseases were either common sources or host to host epidemics. Various microbes were participating as cholera, influenza, syphilis, malaria, typhus, smallpox and with respect to children measles and mumps. The "black death" was a major infectious disease which persecuted European people, especially in the years 1346–1353. These threats have been brought under control through medicinal progress, but they are breaking out again surprisingly as the example of HIV shows.

Famines caused many millions of fatalities in Medieval Europe, they were familiar occurrences which laid to its most dramatic crisis in the Great Famine from 1315 to 1317 (Watkins and Menken 1985). Bad weather with continuing rain and cool were followed by crop failures and missing fodder for the life-stock and finally the nutrition for the broad population broke down. A dramatic reduction of the average life expectation happened and nutrition was sometimes restricted to wealthy people. This threat has been overcome in Europe—not elsewhere in the world—by improving harvest and food production.

Witch-hunting was a method of killing innocent people. The hunting of witches happened during long times of the Middle Ages from about 450 and 1750, but special cases are virulent up today (**Levack B. P.**). Economic advantages and religious motives were in the background. According to guesses 40,000 people or more were victims of witch-hunting among them mostly women. The method was to accuse individuals for religious reasons to be related to the devil and to kill them cruel through fire and torture. Witch-hunting in this amount lost it's acceptance in the secularized world.

In modern times, different sources are responsible for permanent fatalities. Two examples for modern death tolls, which are morally very different, are traffic fatalities and suicides.

Traffic fatalities add up yearly to about 30,000 road deaths. Such a number of people were killed yearly on EU-roads. Interestingly, the road deaths are often perceived by the people as an unavoidable and undramatic by-product of traffic, which are caused by the people itself. Fortunately, there is a decreasing tendency for road deaths in the past decades.[4]

Suicides are another area, where stable amount of fatalities happen each year in Europe and its countries. Due to intentional self-harm in Europe in the year 2016 around 58,000 people have passed according to the World Health Report, among them many more males than females. As the WHO tells, *Europe* is the most suicidal continent in the entire world.[5] This may seem paradoxical with respect to the high level of life satisfaction which is always found for Europe. But we have to take into account that suicide and satisfaction have different causes. Suicide may happen despite a high satisfaction of a population and dissatisfied people may resist to suicide. Suicide research hints to its own causes for this decision.

The societies in Europe of the past millenniums were exposed to wars and conflicts as well as to plagues and epidemics. During a long time, they were unable to cope with these challenges but in the course of time they attained some progress in fighting diseases and infections though threats remained in every life (http://www.de.com/item_90608.aspx). But plagues and epidemics were brought under control to a high degree.[6]

Also the wartimes were reduced after the two World Wars. But not "peace" moreover the term "Cold War" came up to design the character of the new period. The so-called Cold War was a time of hostile relationships between the Warsaw Pact (Soviet Union and its Satellite states) and the NATO (USA and Allies). The division of Europe into East and West is closely connected with the Cold War, and it is a time of reduced security and well-being but a time without severe war-burdens. Despite hostile relationships, the time from 1947 to 1990 was without great wars between European peoples, which is regarded as a success of the European Unification. This is a contribution to the well-being of people who lost less of their people than in the earlier times.

As a result of the World War II, the Warsaw Pact was created and penetrated somewhat into the western half of Europe, including Poland, Czechoslovakia, Romania and Bulgaria. The change came during the Peaceful Revolution of 1990, which was followed by the inclusion of significant parts of Eastern Europe into the European Union (for example the Baltic states, Poland, Romania, Bulgaria and others).

---

[4]http://sofiaglobe.com/2017/03/29/bulgaria-had-highest-road-accident-death-rate-in-the-eu-in-2016-official/.

[5]https://www.google.de/search?source=hp&q=suicide+in+Europe+WHO&oq=suicide+in+Europe+WHO&gs_.

[6]A number of regional conflicts within European countries were during the Cold War virulent through many years, including Basque's country, North Ireland, South Tyrol and the Balkans. But the number of war deads went down in the course of time.

Interestingly, there is no registration of peacetimes as we find it for wartimes. But also peace is regarded in the long view "peace from the Antique up to day'. Most attention to peace is given to peace-making and peace contracts (Arnold 2018). The contribution of peace contracts to the well-being of the people is not to overstate. The Treaty of Westphalia, which ended the Thirty Years' War in 1648 was one of the most important. Modern societies could learn from the historical examples of the successful finishing of wars. "Make Love not War" was the universal slogan of people in support of the peacemakers struggle for well-being.

References

Bös, M., & Rosenbrock, H. (2015). Wars and violence through the centuries. In W. Glatzer, L. Camfield, V. Moller, & M. Rojas (Eds.), *Global handbook of quality of life*. Dordrecht: Springer.

Müller, M. (Ed.). (2018). *Picasso – Von den Schrecken des Krieges zur Friedenstaube (Picasso – From the threats of the war to the peace of dove)*. Münster: Sandstein-Verlag.

Watkins, S.C., Menken, J. (1985). Famines in historical perspective. *In Population and Development Review*, 11(4) pp 647–675

Chapter 6
Long-Term State- and Nation-Building in Europe

Abstract Beginning of Europe modern state structures can be recognized in the past millennium. Some kingdoms existing already around 1000 CE are now modern nation-states. State- and nation-building were a long-term process in which national-state were formed with clear boundaries, uniform administration, defined citizen rights and so on. It took the time into the 1950s to build from the isolated national state the supranational unit of the European Union. The process of state- and nation-building did not aim at homogenous states which offer a similar level of well-being to its citizens. Europeans attained rather high levels of well-being in global comparisons. Heterogeneity is found in all the national measures from the economic accounts (GDP), satisfaction with life (SWL), Human Development Index (HDI) and social progress (WISP). The leading question is if Europe can be described as a continent of variety or a continent of inequality.

The European states and nations have always exposed their people in a characteristic manner to certain components of quality of life, sometimes more positive sometimes extremely negative. The nations of Europe constituted a hierarchy of higher and lower levels of well-being which was rather stable over time. Depending on citizenship, somebody who belonged to Denmark had continually much higher chance to participate at quality of life than somebody from Bulgaria.[1]

The political map of Europe is composed of states which have emerged in the last millennium, some very early and others in the recent centuries (Parker 1994). According to historians, the state structure of today was one millennium ago resembling at the horizon. At this time, kingdoms were prevailing which were later transformed to nation-states. State- and nation-building[2] in Europe were a long-during process in which the decision was made who was citizen of which nation (Held 1996). In

---

[1] This is documented using three indicators for all the EU countries at the end of this chapter.

[2] State formation is a historical process which ended up with the establishment of a central authority (government) and an administrative infrastructure (state bureaucracy) that gained control over a territory and was able to defend its borders. In addition nation-building was focused on the sociopolitical integration of peoples and the development of a national identity on the basis of a common history, common language and common values.

© The Author(s), under exclusive licence to Springer Nature Switzerland AG 2019
W. Glatzer, *History and Politics of Well-Being in Europe*, SpringerBriefs in Well-Being and Quality of Life Research, https://doi.org/10.1007/978-3-030-05048-1_6

the course of state- and nation-building (Rokkan 1975), people[3] were assorted to territories which were the basis for their experience of quality of life.

At the beginning of the past two millenniums stood the Roman Empire around the Mediterranean Sea with its centre in Southern Europe. The fall of the Western Roman Empire at 476 BE was accompanied by a successive reorganization of the settlements of many European peoples. After the end of the Roman Empire, the "Germanic migration period" changed peoples and territories. During three centuries, many Germanic tribes participated in comprehensive long-distance migration processes among them the Goths, the Vandals, the Anglo-Saxons, the Alamanni, the Franks and some others. When the "Völkerwanderung", as it is called in German, came to an end, the regional distribution of the Germanic tribes was rather different from the beginning of the migration period. Interesting that deficits of well-being are often regarded as a reason for the migration waves.[4] In the centuries after the Germanic migration, the dramatic change of state structures was going on. It was the dynasty of the Merovingians who unified large territories of the fragmented Europe under the rule of Christianity. Their heritage was further developed to the Frankish Empire of Charlemagne (768–814) which constituted the only kingdom that is today regarded as a predecessor of an unified Europe (Parker 1994, p. 106). It is an often repeated statement that Charlemagne has brought prosperity to his people.[5] Charlemagne has been regarded as the "Father of Europe" (*Pater Europae*), as he united most of Western Europe for the first time.[6] Main borders of his empire were in the South-West the mountain range of the Pyrenees, which separated the "Mohammedans" and in the North-East the river "Elbe" which constituted the border to the East-European Slavs. In this constellation, the idea of a unified Europe emerged.

When Charlemagne distributed his empire among his sons, this was the beginning of a more than thousand years during process of dissolving Europe into middle-sized and small territories, mostly having the constitution of a kingdom (Fig. 6.1).

Around the millennium change of the year 1000, which means 1000 years ago, there existed the kingdoms of England (later Great Britain) and France, also the kingdoms of Sweden and Norway (Black 2005). Altogether there countries have a history of about 1000 years with moderate changes. On the historical map of 1000 CE, we find aside of these stable kingdoms additional the kingdoms of Poland and Hungary, which were growing and shrinking in the course of centuries. And about 500 years later, there are the kingdoms of Spain, Portugal, Scotland, Denmark, the Netherlands, Ireland and the Czarist Empire of Russia. This long destiny of the European kingdoms constitutes a historical power. They transformed their inner

---

[3]A similar perspective on state- and nation-building Europe is used in Held (1996).

[4]But other causes of the big European migrations are also debated, for example, the migration pressure from the Huns who came from the East.

[5]It is also often told that he brought peace, but this is usually restricted to the inside of his country, whereas at the borders he fought many wars.

[6]According to historical research, the time of Charlemagne is described as a betterment of the historical trouble before, and especially administrative procedures have been adapted in Europe which enforced the homogeneity of religious and living conditions in Europe.

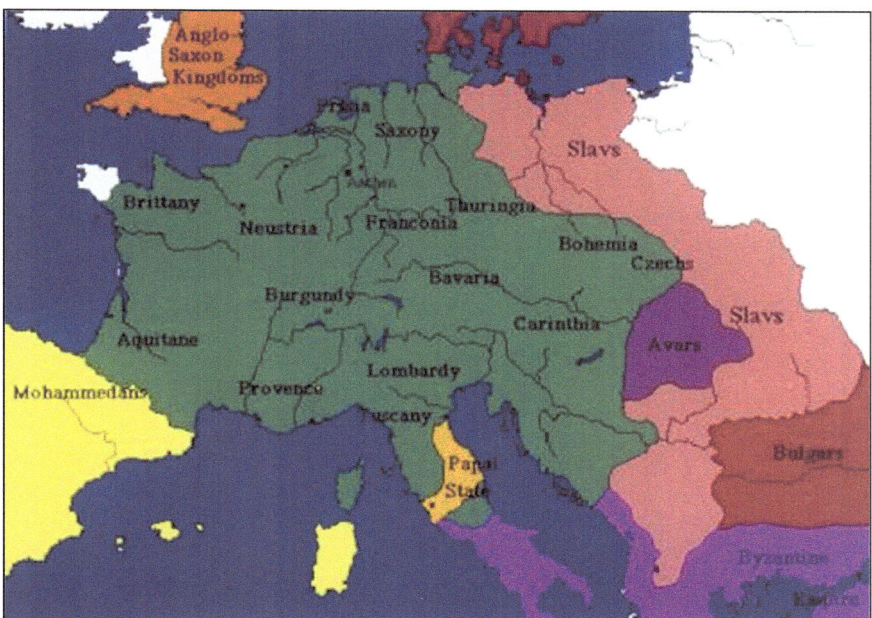

Fig. 6.1 Frankish Empire of Charlemagne around 800. *Source* https://www.awesomestor es.com/asset/view/Frankish-Holy-Roman-Empire-of-Charlemagne-Map

constitutions, but they constituted through the centuries up today stable elements of the European state structure (Maddison 2001).

In contrast to this continuity stood the fragmented territories of Italy and especially in Germany. Italy remained separated into a number of sub-states until 1861. German territories were known for their "*Kleinstaaterei*" *(territorial augmentation)*, a proliferation of small states in Central Europe. In earlier centuries, Germany alone consisted of 300 territorial units. Modern Germany, which is now the largest state in the EU, was formed in 1871 by unifying 39 states under Prussian leadership. Thus, Germany was the delayed country in Europe which performed in the last century the task of state- and nation-building. But the foundation of new states went on after the Balkan War in 2005 when five states gained independence.

Europe grew historically to 48 nations of rather different size[7] and structure. Especially after World War II, unifying endeavours took place, which resulted mainly in two organizations, in the European Council since 1951 (European Council 2011), containing 48 *European states and the European Union* including today 28 member states since 1956.[8] The European Union began with six founding members from

---

[7]Part of the EU are also the outermost countries which belong to an EU mainland as there are the Azores and Madeira (Portugal), Canary Islands (Spain), French Guyana (France) and some others.

[8]The status of applicant for the European Union has a number of countries, especially on the Balkans.

Western Europe[9] and grew stepwise until its enlargement with nine countries from Eastern Europe in 2004 (see Fig. 6.2).

The EU Member States are from the various areas of the continent and of different size (Gerhards and Lengfeld 2015). They include in (2008):

Northern Europe with Denmark (5.7), Finland (5.5), Sweden (9.9);

Central Europe with Germany (80.6), Poland (38.6), Czech Republic (10.6), Hungary (9.8), Austria (8.6), Slovakia (5.4), Slovenia (2.0);

Western Europe with Great Britain (65.5), France (64.9), the Netherlands (17.0), Belgium (11.4), Ireland (4.7), Luxembourg (0.6);

Southern Europe with Italy (59.8), Spain (46.8), Greece (10.9), Portugal (10.3), Cyprus (1.2), Malta (0.4);

The South-East of Europe with Romania (19.2), Bulgaria (7.0) and Croatia (4.2);

North-East Europe, the Baltic countries with Lithuania (2.8), Latvia (1.9) and Estonia (1.3) (Fig. 6.3).

Less than half of the European states have remained outside the European Union, and prosperous and mighty states are among them. Outside the European Union in Western Europe are Switzerland (8.4), Norway (5.3) and Iceland (0.3). People of Great Britain decided in a Brexit vote to leave the EU, and the government is still engaged in negotiations with the EU. On the other side in South-Eastern Europe,

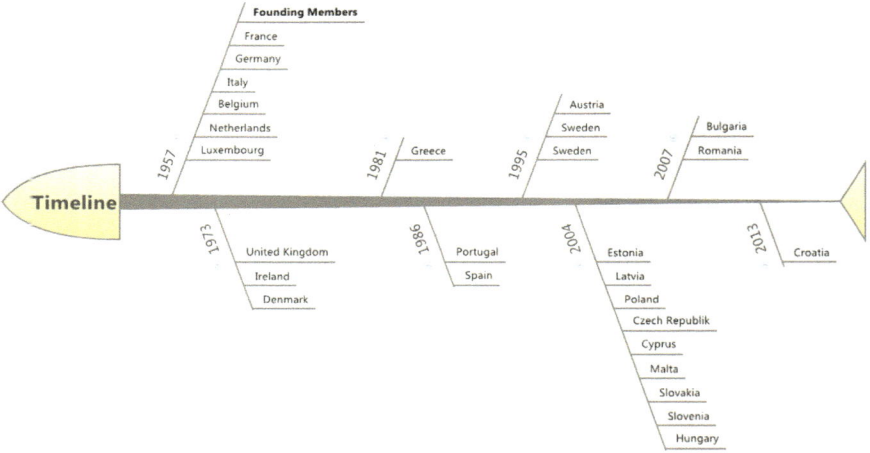

Fig. 6.2 Ongoing European enlargement—founding members and joining members in the European Union. *Source* European Union (2015); construction from Kolja Glatzer

---

[9]The EU has been built on predecessors and accompanying institutions. The "European Coal and Steel Organization" was a first important step for European cooperation which led into several EU treatises. Aside, the "European Council", founded in 1951, included all European countries but implemented weaker forms of integration than the EU. A common European currency—the Euro—was introduced in 2007 in 15 member countries and constituted a further step of European integration.

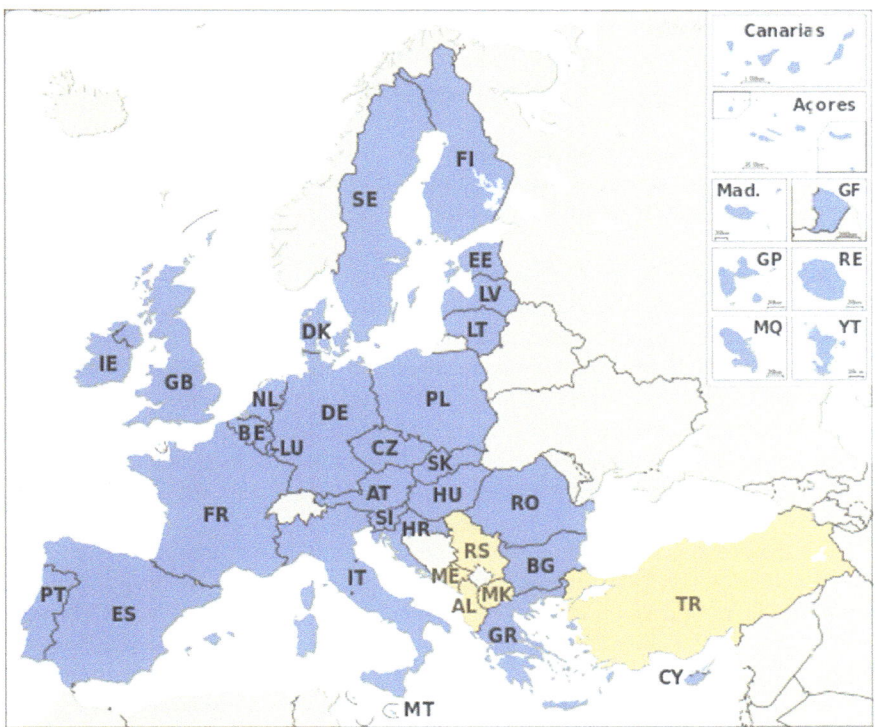

Fig. 6.3 Nation-states in Europe according to EU membership, EU candidate countries, non-members of EU. *Notes* EU members = blue; non-EU members = grey; candidates for EU membership = yellow. *Source* http://de.wikipedia.org/wiki/Datei:EU_Member_states_and_Candidate_countries_map.svg

possible EU candidates are on the Balkans, namely Serbia (8.8), Kosovo (3.8), Bosnia and Herzegovina (3.8), Albania (2.9), Macedonia (2.1), Kosovo (1.8), Montenegro (0.6). The remaining, geographically rather large part outside the European Union in Eastern Europe, are Russia (143.4), Ukraine (44.4), Belarus (9.5), Moldova (4.0); Also a small part of Turkey in the West of the Bosporus is in European territory.

The EU states constitute 28 nations which differ extremely in territorial size and the number of citizens and last but not least in centuries of their existence. Also important is that Europeans states have developed to very different types of economies and societies (Gerhards and Lengfeld 2015). To characterize the European societies, a number of indicators are available which are worldwide used.

The GDP: the Gross Domestic Product is a conventional measure for national economic performance derived from the economic accounts; it is a single indicator for a complex construct (World Bank 2017).

The SWL: the satisfaction with life is a subjective measure, which is worldwide used in representative country surveys, and it is related to the subjective state of the nation in the eyes of the people. SWL is a pure subjective measure depending on the perception of the people, whereas the GDP is designed as an objective measure depending on the rules of economic accounting (European Union 2017; Helliwell 2018).

The HDI: the Human Development Index has been developed in the context of the United Nations and presents a quantification of human development above economic measures. It is oriented towards health, education and living standard (United Nations 2016).

The WISP: the concept of "social progress" is grounded in philosophy and is built as a multi-dimensional indicator since some decades including all regions and nearly all countries of the world. Its content is expressed in the composite WISP indicator which is derived from eight areas with sub-indexes and 40 basic indicators (Estes 1988). The subareas are education, health status, women status, defence effort, economic status, demography, environmental, social chaos, cultural diversity and welfare effort. Each sub-index is the result of a number of basic indicators, and all the indices combined together are resulting in one WISP Score, the Weighted Index for Social Progress.

Each European country has a special position in the European rank order. The objective indicator of GDP and the subjective indicator of SWL are resulting in two somewhat different rank orders, but they are showing the same tendency. Denmark, Finland and Sweden have the best values for satisfaction with life; Latvia, Bulgaria and Greece have the lowest values. Economically are at the top Luxembourg, Ireland and Denmark and at the bottom Bulgaria, Romania and Poland. With respect to GDP, it makes sense to speak of inequality; with respect to SWL, the picture is of diversity (Fig. 6.4).

The traditional indicator for economic performance is the Gross Domestic Product measured regularly within the economic accounts (World Bank 2017). The GDP per

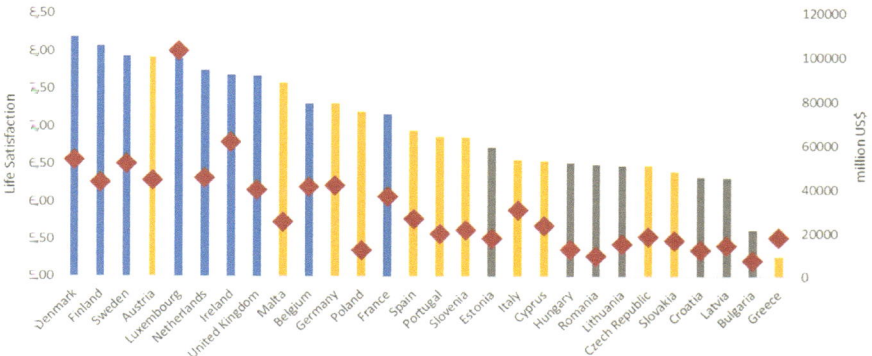

Fig. 6.4 Measurements of economic performance and subjective well-being in EU states in 2016: Gross Domestic Product per capita and average life satisfaction. *Source* European Union (2017). Eurofound Quality of Life Survey 2016. World Bank (2017) GDP per capita in current US$; Construction from Kolja Glatzer

capita attains in the EU highest values—also worldwide—especially in Luxembourg (103.2 $) followed by Ireland (62.6) and Denmark (53.7). Within the EU, the poorest countries in terms of GDP are Bulgaria (7.4), Romania (9.5) and Poland (12.3). There are indicated huge differences of the GDP per capita between Bulgaria and Luxembourg—Luxembourg is 15 times higher—and the difference of Denmark and Poland—Denmark is eight times higher. Due to these huge GDP differences, the economic well-being of people in Europe is characterized by inequality.

The average life satisfaction (ALS) in Europe lays on the ten-point scale from one to ten between 7.5 for Denmark and 4.7 for Bulgaria (European Union 2017).[10] Finland and the Netherlands have also high life satisfaction, and Portugal and Greece have beside Bulgaria the lowest life satisfaction. This difference is rather high as far as we have experience with country comparisons using the satisfaction scale.

The differences of the Human Development Index (United Nations 2016) in the EU countries are also strong. The empirical range of the Human Development Index in EU countries runs from 0.926 (Germany) to 0.794 (Bulgaria) which means officially "very high human development" for Germany and as the only European country in the second category "high human development" for Bulgaria. There is no European country which is designed as "medium development" which gives an impression of Europe's level in the world economy. The top of the HDI ladder are beside Germany (0.926) constituted by Denmark (0.925) and the Netherlands (0.924), altogether are situated in Central and Northern Europe. The low countries in the EU are beside Bulgaria (0.794), Romania (0.802) and Croatia (0.827), altogether situated in the South-East of Europe. As the sub-components of the HDI index shows, the differences in health, education and living standards contribute to these inequalities.

Another construction from the university context is the Weighted Index for Social Progress. Among the twenty-five highest performing countries, there are 20 countries from Europe which is an outstanding result (Estes 2018). Denmark is the highest, and Greece is the lowest. European's country performance is not unique but excellent. The countries abroad which are comparable with most European countries are Japan, Iceland, New Zealand, Australia, and Canada. Though the WISP indicators in Asia and Africa show higher advancement than in Europe, it is difficult for these areas to attain the European level. Europe was a pioneer continent whose paths were followed soon by some other peoples—more or less—and by others not.

In the average of the three indicators GDP, HDI and ALS, representing economic success, human development and satisfaction with life, the country of Denmark is on position 1 and Bulgaria is on position 28. There is a tendency to attain similar positions in all the three societal dimensions. Above there is a regional cleavage;

---

[10]In the year 2016, in European countries, two supranational representative survey sets were carried through, one by Eurofound and one by the World Happiness Study. Whereas in the Eurofound survey, the simple satisfaction ladder from 1 to 10 was implemented; the World Happiness Survey adapted the Cantril ladder, which is somewhat more complicate. According to the results, the life satisfaction values of both surveys differ somewhat in detail but not in the main tendency Top and bottom countries tend to be the same in both surveys. It is no-good solution that different scales for life satisfaction are used in the various surveys and that, therefore, no precise comparability of the results exists.

Northern and Western states are at the top of economic success, human development and life satisfaction, and Southern and Eastern states constitute the low area of well-being.

At the actual level of state- and nation-building, there exists a picture of heterogeneity. Heterogeneity between countries is visible with respect to the size of nations, with respect to the duration of country's existence, with respect to national economic success and to human development goals and finally to life satisfaction. Instead of a homogeneity of states, there is a multi-variety of states on different levels of success (Fig. 6.4). Access to more or less better levels is given by citizenship. Only the citizen of a country has the right in civic, economic and political respects to use the resources of the country. A European citizenship would create more equality, but some differences would still exist.

All the indicators which are in use for measuring the well-being of societies contain the problem that the final results depend not only on the characteristics of the societies but also on the values which constitute the basis for the indicator construction.

References

Black, J. (2005). *Dumont Atlas of world history*. London: Dorling Kindersley.
Council of Europe. (2011). *Towards a Europe of shared social responsibilities: Challenges and strategies*. Strasbourg.
European Union. (2015). *Quality of life—Facts and views*. Eurostat, Statistical Books.
European Union. (2017). *Eurofound quality of life survey 2016*. Dublin.
Estes, R. J. (1988). *Trends in world social development. The Social Progress of Nations, 1970–1987*. New York/Westport/London: Praeger.
Estes, R. J. (2018). *The social progress of nations revisited, 1970–2018: A half century of promise and progress*. Manuscript to be published in Social Indicators Research 2018.
Gerhards, J., & Lengfeld, H. (2015). *European citizenship and social integration in the European Union*. London: Routledge.
Hall, S., Held, D., Hubert, D., & Thompson, K. (1996). Modernity. *An Introduction to Modern Societies*. Massachusetts: Blackwell Publisher pp. 55–90.
Helliwell, J. F., Layard, H., & Sachs, J. D. (2018). *World Happiness Report 2018*.
Maddison, A. (2001). *The world economy. A millenial perspective*. Paris: OECD.
Parker, G. (1994). *The time atlas of world history*. London: Times Books.
Rokkan, S. (1975). Dimensions of state formation and nation-building: A possible paradigm for research on variations within Europe, pp. 562–600. In C. Tilly (Ed.), (1975) *The formation of National States in Western Europe*. Princeton N. J.: Princeton University Press.
United Nations. (2016). *Human Development Report 2016*.
World Bank. (2017). *GDP per Capita in current US $*. https://data.worldbank.org/indicator/NY.GDP.PCAP.CD?locations=SL.

Chapter 7
Economic Growth and Levels of Living

Abstract After some millennia of relative economic stagnation, an increasing living standard was enabled since the nineteenth century by the success of industrialization. Economic growth was different by countries but has been improving the living standard in all countries. But after two centuries of economic progress in Europe, the over-optimistic material aspirations of the past were not fulfilled. Despite increasing income levels, there remained a severe burden from poverty, as defined by experts, and of subjectively felt scarcity, as ordinary people define their economic situation. Above economic growth was joined by ecological and climate threats. People in the European Union, especially the younger ones, have to worry about their future life chances.

Long-term Economic Development. Beside Europeans demographic enlargement in close connection a unique socio-economic rise happened, which is described as follows: It begun from a low level of development and took an exceptional growth.

> "By the year 1000, its (Europeans) income levels had fallen below those in Asia and North Africa. In its lengthy resurrection, it caught up with China (the world leader) in the fourteenth century. By 1820, its levels of income and productivity were measured more than twice as high as in the rest of the world. By 1913, the income level in Western Europa and in Western Offshoots was more than six times that in the rest of the world" (Maddison 2001 p. 49). [1]

The rise of Europe depended significantly on Europeans own innovations and performance though critical notes state also an exploiting behaviour "Western economy advance also involved devastating wars and beggar-your-neighbour policies"

---

[1] It should not be overseen that this development did not happen straightforward it was moreover often broken by wars, crisis, plagues, epidemics, famines and disasters. In general, social development was always characterized by ups and downs and by crisis and boom-times.

(Maddison 2001 p. 49). Europe's growing prosperity was assisted by the exploitation of colonies which happened through some centuries and came to an end after World War I. At this time, Europe began to lose its globally leading position, which was developed in the millennium before. Europe's share of world GDP grew historically from 17.9% in 1500 to 33.6% in 1913 and documents that Europe gained economic world dominance. The reconstruction of the long-term economic development of Europe indicates its exceptional prosperity in this time. But after World War I it lost its prior position and was shrinking to 20.6% of world's GDP in 1998 (Maddison 2001, p. 127).

Historically, economic growth is the foundation of an improvement of the economic conditions of life and an increase of levels of living. It is globally unique how the European continent increased economic growth in the last two centuries (Flora et al. 1987). The innovative way into industrialization and succeeding post-industrialization was taken after two millennia of relative stagnation. Advances in technology and productivity opened a new development path into the nineteenth century (Fig. 6.3). This economic growth, which was previously unknown, was attained by more and more countries (World Bank, 2010).

European countries took a speedway from 1820 onward and some of its countries grew extremely after World War II (Olson 1982). As Fig. 7.1 documents England was the "motherland" of industrialization and leads therefore with respect to economic growth. Followers came first from West European countries as the Netherlands and Sweden, but finally countries from all around the world joined the industrial path. Germany, which was a latecomer of industrialization, laid behind the Netherlands, Sweden and France, but recovered quickly in a so-called economic miracle from the breakdown in the World War II. Italy and Spain as examples from Southern Europe attained typically a relative lower economic growth. Finally Poland, as an example of the Eastern Europe countries, had from the beginning of industrialization a much lower GDP per capita. But some economic growth has emerged earlier or later in all European countries and this was so impressive that many people expected to overcome scarcity and to run into a luxurious future.

Document VI: Historical Promises of Expected Affluence in the nineteenth Century

"The authors of the nineteenth century had promised to the people the end of scarcity with such a supply of goods, that they were able without counting that they could live according to fun and joy to afford everything to live joyful with another" (Bell 1973 p. 360).

As it is obvious today this luxury stage of well-being was never attained. The historic accomplishments were missed though the economic progress in the last century was tremendously. Nevertheless according to expert descriptions household equipment and every-day life changed fundamentally in the past century.

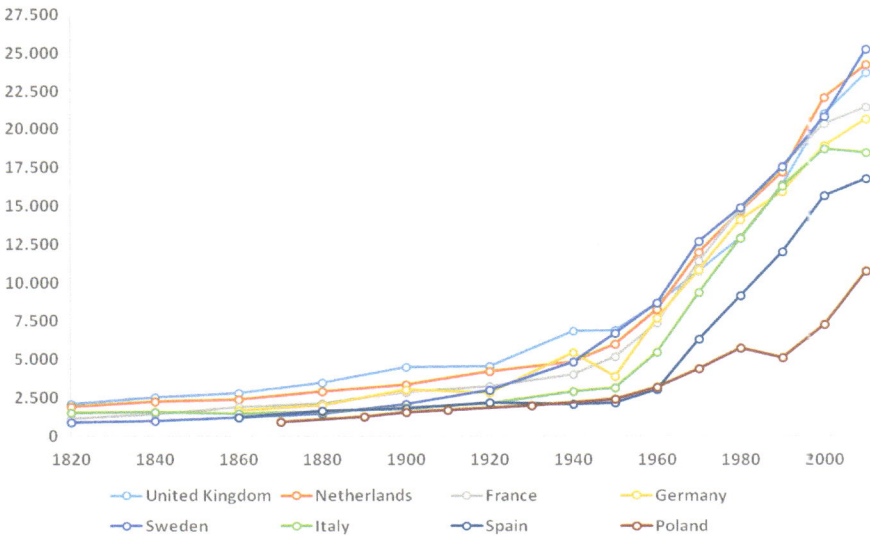

Fig. 7.1 Gross domestic product per capita in selected countries of Europe from 1820 to 2010. *Source* Van Zanden et al. (2014), p. 67

Document VII: The transformation of every-day life equipment in Europe during the past century

"The amenities of life, that almost all of us take for granted today including electricity, indoor plumbing, safe public water and sewage systems, instant mass communications, access to technologically sophisticated medical care, a remarkable variety of fresh and indigenously packaged food from around the nation and the world, free public education, low infant mortality, and long life expectancy were virtually absent one century ago" (De Jong 2015, p. 45).

Everyday life of broad segments of the European population has changed fundamentally from a poor to a more amenable life. Nobody is old enough to know these changes from own experience because nobody remembers how life was before one's life. There has been established a basic inventory for the needs of most people[2] but above there developed a broad differentiation of income and goods, which were available for many but not available for all.

Subjective perception of levels of living. It is impossible to decide if the subjective construction of reality is more or less important than the objective construction of reality. Society are always stratified and scientific experts may construct another stratification than the people have in their mind. The subjective definition of one's level of living is well expressed in the answers of the question about the ability to make ends meet. It gives a clear picture of the stratification of European society in the eyes of European people. Though the question does not use the term poverty, it

---

[2]One population category, the homeless people, is by far excluded from these basic amenities. There life in Europe is not very well known.

seems to be a reasonable socio-economic poverty measure. People who define their ability to make ends meet "with difficulty" or "with great difficulty" are regarded in the risk of poverty.

The answer categories to the make ends meet question offers six levels which are running from "great difficulties" to "very easily". In Europe the question, how people feel about their socio-economic conditions of their household, is used since a longer time in different surveys. Their result is that economic progress has not only attained small groups of the population moreover the broad middle of the population, grew to a historical unknown prosperity (Fig. 7.2).

The percentages of European people, who have different abilities to make ends meet with their household budget, show a socio-economic stratification of European people which is a mixture of prosperity and poverty, but prosperity is overwhelming. There are some percentages of prosperity at the top of 10% (making ends meet very easily) and of poverty at the bottom (making ends meet with great difficulty) in an amount of 6%. Difficulties are reported from 9% of the adult Europeans, which is also a risk of poverty. A broad majority of the population defines its household situation in the middle which includes easily (22%), fairly easily (30%) and with some difficulty (28%). Parts of the population belong to the middle class, if they are below the top 10% on the one side and above the population group who has difficulties or strong difficulties to make ends meet on the other side.

Altogether 76% of the European people have the opinion to exist in the middle of the levels of living, they do not have affluence and they do not have severe difficulties to make ends meet. The European population is a stable broad middle-class society accompanied by with a small prosperous class above the middle class and two smaller classes in the risk of poverty below the middle class. But the volume of the middle class varies in the EU Member States. It is above 76% in 20 of the member states and it is lowest in Greece, Romania, and Bulgaria and Croatia, where small middle classes

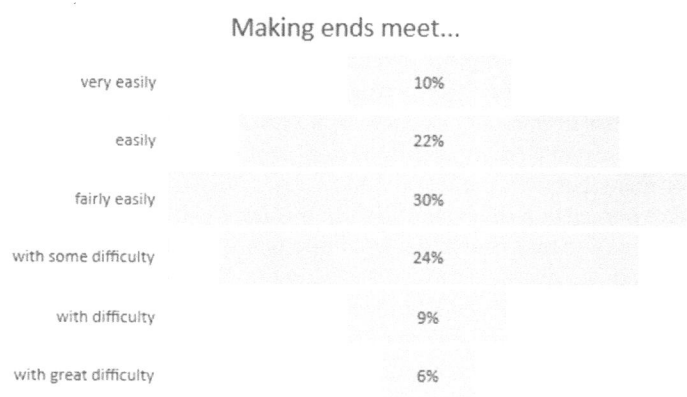

Fig. 7.2 Abilities of European people to make ends meet in 2016. *Source* Data received from Eurofound (2018), own construction

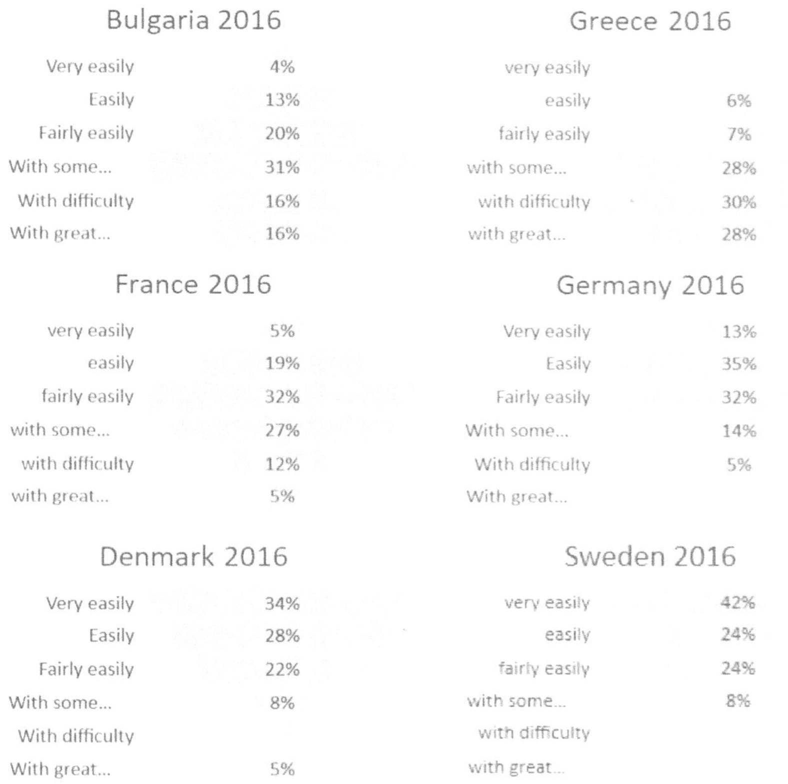

Bulgaria 2016

Very easily	4%
Easily	13%
Fairly easily	20%
With some...	31%
With difficulty	16%
With great...	16%

Greece 2016

very easily	
easily	6%
fairly easily	7%
with some...	28%
with difficulty	30%
with great...	28%

France 2016

very easily	5%
easily	19%
fairly easily	32%
with some...	27%
with difficulty	12%
with great...	5%

Germany 2016

Very easily	13%
Easily	35%
Fairly easily	32%
With some...	14%
With difficulty	5%
With great...	

Denmark 2016

Very easily	34%
Easily	28%
Fairly easily	22%
With some...	8%
With difficulty	
With great...	5%

Sweden 2016

very easily	42%
easily	24%
fairly easily	24%
with some...	8%
with difficulty	
with great...	

Fig. 7.3 Stratifcation of levels of living in selected European countries: Bulgaria and Greece, Germany and France, Denmark and Sweden. *Source* Data received from Eurofound (2018), own construction

in the sense of making ends meet exist. The countries in Europe are subjectively very different types of societies. We find poverty-grounded societies in Bulgaria and Greece, a strong middle class in Germany and France and a top-level society in Denmark and Sweden (Fig. 7.3).

Bulgaria and Greece are less developed early industrial societies, where most people are on a middle level of living but relatively strong shares of people are on the lowest level of existence. Much more people are on the two lower levels of living than on the two upper levels. In these societies, the fight against poverty is a prevalent task.

Germany and France present societies, where the subjectively perceived level of living is fully developed and the stratification system looks like an onion standing on the top. Most people are on upper levels and the top level contains more people than the two lowest levels. France is not so developed as the more prosperous Germany.

Denmark and Sweden are post-industrial societies where the upper two levels of living include the majority of the population. On the level of living in the middle strata are more people than on the lower strata. All in all the picture looks like a pyramid standing on the top. It could be that living with great difficulties in a prosperous society is harder than to live among a broader number of poor people in a medium society.

The risk of poverty. How far poverty has been overcome historically is often in dispute. The discussion is associated with the core problem that the style and height of poverty measures was controversial (Atkinson 1998). Poverty is a term based on conventions, values and preferences and there are different levels of living which are regarded as poverty. Because opinions about poverty are so different the answer of poverty experts was to speak of the risk of poverty instead of postulating an existing poverty. It makes no significant difference if governments fight against poverty or against the risk of poverty. It is most important to mention that there was a declaration of the European Union for a social inclusion target to lift some millions of people out of the risk of poverty and social exclusion. At risk of poverty or social exclusion is defined as a situation of people which have either a monetary risk of poverty[3] or they are severely materially deprived[4] or they are living in a household with a very low work intensity. An advantage of this risk-of poverty-rate is a certain amount of official recognition.

According to poverty studies in times before Europeans industrialization, the majority of the European population lived in poverty. After two hundred years of industrialization and economic growth, there remained according to the risk-of-poverty and social exclusion a share in the amount of 23.7% of the European adult population. Social state transfers play a major role to keep the poverty rate at this level in the EU. But the poverty rates are very different in the various EU countries and the burden for the people varies a lot (Fig. 7.4).

Relatively, high poverty rates are present in Bulgaria (41.3%), Romania (37.4%), Greece (35.7%), Latvia (30.5) which are all above 30% and constitute main challenges for the countries. Czech Republic (14.0%), Sweden (16.0%), the Netherlands (16.4%) and Finland (16.7) have the lowest relative poverty rate below 17%. It indicates that they have reduced the risk of poverty in their countries with some success. Twenty-two EU Member States show a poverty rate between 30 and 17% and at this point of time this is the prevailing level for monetary poverty and social exclusion given the 60% distance to mean income.

---

[3] The at-risk of-poverty rate is the share of people with an equivalized disposable income (after social transfers) below the threshold which is set at 60% of the national median equivalized disposable income after social transfers.

[4] In terms of goods, which are missed in the poor households, poverty is defined as a deficit of four household goods from ten: Mortgage or rent payments … or other loan payments. One week holiday away from home. Meal with meat, chicken, fish or vegetarian equivalent every second day. Unexpected financial expenses. A telephone (including mobile telephone). A colour TV. A washing machine. A car. Heating to keep the home adequately warm. The survey result is that 6% of European adult people are missing at least four of these goods and they are therefore classified as severely deprived.

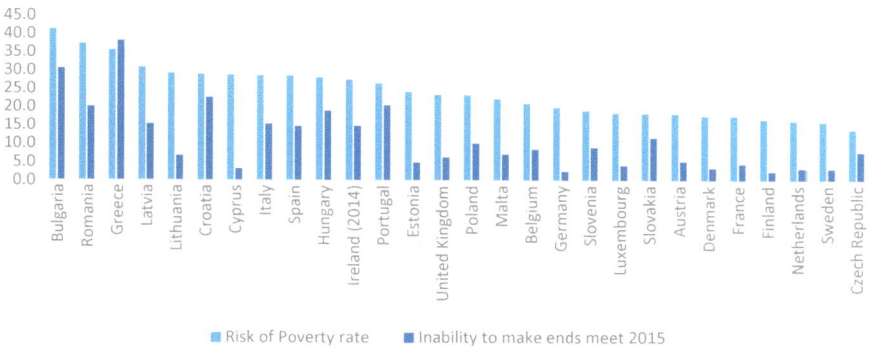

Fig. 7.4 Risk-of-poverty rate and share of people, who have difficulties to make ends meet in Europe in the year 2015. *Sources* http://appsso.eurostat.ec.europa.eu/nui/show.do?dataset= ilc_mdes09&lang=en, http://ec.europa.eu/eurostat/statistics-explained/index.php/people_at_risk_ of_poverty_or_social_exclusion

The populations of Finland, Germany and Sweden report the lowest shares of self-perceived "poor" people. On the other side, the populations of Bulgaria and Romania and Greece indicate that they have the most difficulties. Some successful countries are close to the goal of a satisfying income distribution—only 3% feel themselves poor—whereas the other countries with about 20% feeling poor are far away from this goal. But there is less doubt that the economic growth has created for broad majorities of the European peoples the foundation for a sufficient outcome but the dream of overcoming poverty remained a vision.

The expert definition of the risk of poverty and the subjective definition of the inability to make ends meet are often different. Curiosities are Greece—the only country where the subjective poverty rate is higher than the objective poverty—and Czech Republic—where the objective poverty rate is lowest but the subjective poverty rate is rather high.

Obviously, European people are relieved from the strong poverty pressures of earlier times. In earlier stratification analysis, the picture of the socio-economic stratification was described as an onion which was thick in the middle, thin at the top and somewhat broader towards the bottom. The picture of 2016 is the reverse of this traditional picture. There are more people in the strata at the top then at the bottom. More people express some difficulties. The EU is a middle-class society with a bias to the top.

In the long run, people in Europe were living in an economically growing, structural changing societies which developed from a rural-feudal society through the features of an industrial society to the characteristics of a post-industrial society. The rise of productivity in the course of industrialization brought rising living standards for masses of people but left a lot behind. Prosperity and poverty spread at the same time. Europe's people attained the top of the socio-economic development of the world. More and more countries were attaining similar levels of living. But economic growth has lost its virtue in the process of mass production and mass consumption. Beside inequality and poverty which remained to some degree, ecological threats lead into a "risk society".

References

Atkinson, T. (1998). *Poverty in Europe*. Oxford: Blackwell Publisher.
Bell, D. (1973). *The coming of post-industrial society*. New York: Basic Books.
De Jong, H. (2015). Living standards in a modernizing world. In W. Glatzer, L. Camfield, V. Moller, & M. Rojas (Eds.), (2015). *Global handbook of quality of life*. Dordrecht: Springer.
Eurofound. (2018). *European Union (2017). European Quality of Life survey 2016*. Dublin.
Flora, P., Kraus, F., & Pfenning, W. (1987). *State, economy and society 1815–1975. A data handbook, Vol. II: The growth of industrial societies and capitalist economies*. Frankfurt, Campus/London, Macmillan/Chicago, St. James.
Macdison, A. (2001). *The world economy*. Paris, OECD: A Millennial Perspective.
Olson, M. (1982). *The rise and decline of nations: Economic growth, Stagflation and Social Rigidities*. New Haven and London: Yale University Press.
Van Zanden, J., et al. (Eds.). (2014). *How was life? Global well-being since 1820*. Paris: OECD Publishing.
World Bank. (2010). *The changing wealth of nations*. Washington DC: The World Bank.

Chapter 8
The Spread of Democracy and Their Challenges

Abstract First developed in ancient Greece is the idea of democracy which did not have its breakthrough immediately but was not lost; moreover, it was finally established in many countries of Europe and the world. When the French Revolution in 1789 enforced the demand for democracy, it was the beginning of the spread in European countries. First, the new democracies were incomplete because only men were allowed to participate in elections. Later on, the fight for universal suffrage was decided overall for women. In practice, democracy suffered from unexpected disappointments. Lowering of participation rates happened at national and at supranational elections. People did not develop high trust in the political institutions, and they expressed that they were not much satisfied with the way democracy works. Broad discussion of how democracy could be enforced on national and supranational levels continued.

The pre-modern states in Europe were—far from building democratic constitutions—mostly grounded on absolute or constitutional monarchies. Democratic constitutions spread—starting in 1815—to the Western states of Europe (Flora 1983) and with a long delay to Eastern territories. After two hundred years of democratic development, there are still exceptions of countries in the East, which are resistant to democracy (Canfora 2008).

The way to democracy for European states began with the push of the French Revolution in 1789 to introduce democratic institutions. Since 1815—the first countries were France and Norway—until 1915, the male electorate gained more and more countries and within the countries more and more male people who participated at elections (Flora 1983 p. 91). The rise of democracy seemed a measure to increase peoples influence on their own well-being which was reserved only for men in the nineteenth century. There were high expectations to attain with democratic institutions better and more satisfying living conditions for the citizens (Schaeffer 2015).

There was in the eighteenth century a limitation of suffrage for men which was gradually extended to all adult men before suffrage for women was introduced. Between 1906 (Finland) and 1960 (Cyprus)—joined by France in 1944—countries introduced women suffrage, which had the implication that there were full voting rights for all adult citizens. The breakthrough came with the World War I—and again with World War II—when a bulk of countries generalized enfranchisement and illustrated thus the paradoxical benefits of post-war times. The way into *mass democratization* was finally accompanied by the implementation of parliamentary rules, civil liberties and enfranchisement (Flora 1983). The establishment of suffrage and democratic institutions was for most people a reason for satisfaction and happiness (Fig. 8.1).

Political participation rights, including the right to organize movements, freedom of assembly, and freedom of the press, gave ordinary citizens a voice to express their political demands (Habermas 2011). This situation, in turn, led to the foundation of political parties and stimulated the political mobilization of ever larger parts of the population. Conservative, liberal and socialist social-democratic parties emerged everywhere in Europe, but with different "weights" and in different national constellations and alliances. This explains a lot of the variability in the political history of the European nation-states since the nineteenth century (Fig. 8.2).

After many decades of the implementation of democracy in European nations, the reputation of democracy lost its glamour. Something like the "Veralltäglichung des Charisma" (Max Weber) was breaking through. One main problem is the loss of participation at the elections. As time series since 1990 shows a continual decrease of voter participation that took place with respect to the national elections in European democracies. The participation at elections for the European Parliament was much lower and their decreasing tendency went on. This electoral tiredness was embedded into a diversification of attitudes towards the European democracy (Fig. 8.3) (Council of Europe 2011).

The distance to democracy found its deposit in the trust towards the political system which was not developed sufficiently (Fig. 7.2). The average trust in all countries is rather low, and besides a few high-trust countries, there is a broad majority of low-trust countries. Highest values of trust showed Finland, Malta, Sweden and the Netherlands. The lowest values exist in Portugal, Slovenia and Spain. The average

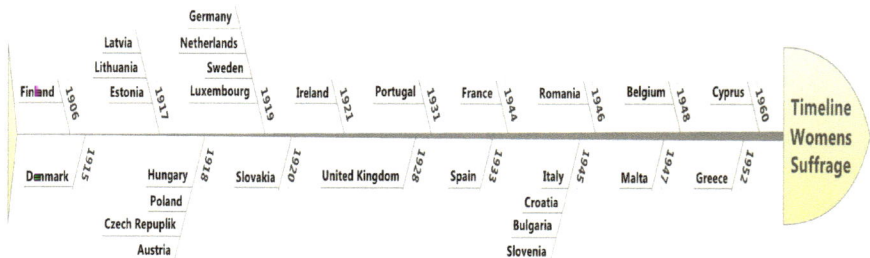

Fig. 8.1 Establishment of women suffrage, respectively, universal suffrage in European states. *Source* Kolja Glatzer according to data of Flora (1983), supplemented by Wikipedia & IPU (http://en.wikipedia.org/wiki/Universal_suffrage and http://www.ipu.org/wmn-e/suffrage.htm)

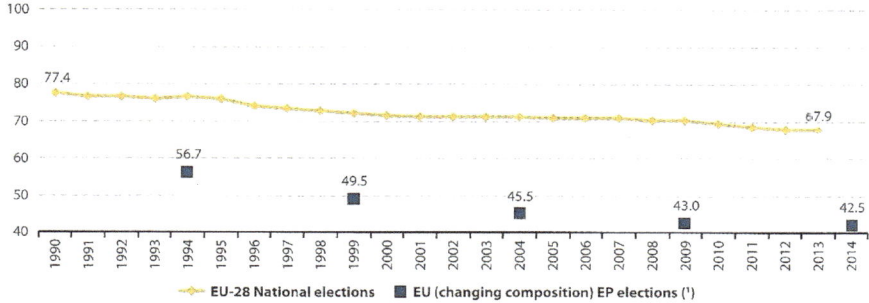

(¹) The figures for EP elections refer to EU composition at the time of the elections, knowing that it has changed considerably since 1994.
Source: Eurostat — International Institute for Democracy and Electoral Assistance (IDEA) Voter turnout database

Fig. 8.2   Voter Turnout in National and EU Parliamentary Elections, 1990–2014[1]. *Source* European Union (2015) p. 192

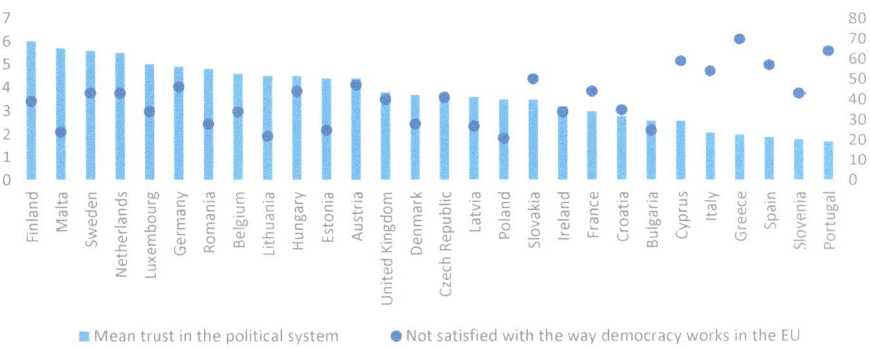

Fig. 8.3   Trust into the political system and satisfaction with the way democracy works in the EU-states 2013. *Data source* European Union (2015) p. 207; OECD (2014)

of trust into the political systems is in the EU low—far below the nominal midpoint of the scale—which is a risk for political stability. There are only few people who would reduce democracy but many people are dissatisfied and would like to improve democracy.

There are further questions for the evaluation of democracies. A standard question is as follows: "How satisfied are you with the way democracy works in your country" (Behr and Braun 2015, p. 138).[1] The question, which is documented in Figure 8.3, is related towards democracy in the European Union. The results, which are measuring a multidimensional attitude, show an astonishingly sceptical attitude against the EU democracy. And there are dramatic differences between Greece, the most critical

---

[1] The authors resume in respect to the democracy question: "As a general evaluation, we would conclude that the satisfaction with the democracy question is not too bad, in a comparative perspective similar multidimensional measurement takes place in all countries".

country towards democracy and Poland, the country with the lowest critic against democracy in the EU.

The way into democracy was in the long run consequent and without realistic alternative, but modern democracy is not self-understanding; it is moreover exposed to challenges and to ongoing tasks to stay alive (Champeau et al 2014, Habermas 2015).

References

Behr, D., & Braun, M. (2015). Satisfaction with the way democracy works: How respondents across countries understand the question. In D. Sztabinski, H. Domanski & F. Sztabinski (Eds.), (2015). *Hopes and anxieties. Six waves of the European Social Survey*. Frankfurt am Main: Lang 121–138.

Canfora, L. (2008). *Democracy in Europe: A history of an ideology*. USA: Wiley.

Champeau, S., Closa, C., Innerarity, D., & Maduro, M. P (Eds.), (2014). *The future of Europe. Democracy, legitimacy and justice after the Euro crisis*. London; New York: Rowman & Littlefield International.

Council of Europe. (2011). *Towards a Europe of shared social responsibilities challenges and strategies*. Strasbourg.

European Union. (2015). *Quality of life—Facts and views*. Eurostat, Statistical Books.

Flora, P. (1983). *State, economy and society in Western Europe 1815–1975. A data handbook, Volume I: The growth of mass democracies and welfare states*. Frankfurt: Campus/London: Macmillan/Chicago: St. James Press.

Habermas, J. (2015). Transnational democracy is necessary and how it is possible. *European Law Journal, 21*(4). https://doi.org/10.1111/eulj.12128.

Habermas, J. (2011) Zur Verfassung Europas—Ein Essay. edition suhrkamp.

Kurunmäki, J., Nevers, J., & te Velde, H. (2018). *Democracy in modern Europe—A conceptual history*. New York, Oxford: Berghahn.

OECD. (2014). Society at a Glance 2014. *OECD Social Indicators*. Paris: OECD Publishing.

Schaeffer, R. K. (2015). The worldwide spread of Democracy. In: W. Glatzer, L. Camfield, V. Moller, & M. Roja (Eds), (2015). *Global handbook of quality of life*. Dordrecht: Springer.

Chapter 9
Emergence and Differentiation of European Welfare States

Abstract Welfare states have always taken over a responsibility for the well-being of the needy people, and in recent times, their task is defined as enabling well-being for all. The engagement of welfare states for the well-being of their people varies in the EU, according to different types of welfare states. Political scientists have assigned to the five types of welfare states "social democratic", "conservative", "liberal", "rudimentary" and "post-socialist". As the main goals of welfare state constitutions are declared sustaining self-sufficiency, reducing the risk of poverty and modifying income distribution. Social-democratic welfare states are most successful with respect to these tasks, and the conservative and liberal are following immediately. High deficits for the well-being of people exist in the rudimentary and post-socialist welfare states.

That collective support is necessary for the assistance of the poor ones was a postulate at the desks of European states already during the Middle Ages and also before. Welfare programmes became institutionalized and constituted a welfare state system that has emerged in European nations at the end of the nineteenth century. In Europe, it was the German social state legislation of 1882 that opened a new phase of societal development which was followed by a growing number of welfare states on European territory. The concept of the welfare state was implemented and differentiated increasingly in Europe's developed nations (Briggs 2000; Bahle et al. 2010).

In the case of the European welfare states, Germany took over the role as pioneer and introduced under its chancellor Bismarck from 1882 to 1889 a number of sociopolitical measures addressed in favour of the working class. They were related to the economic well-being and especially the health of the people and included compulsory insurance for sickness, accidents, invalidity and old age. Later, during the "Weimar Republic" in Germany in 1927 these items were completed by a federal law on unemployment insurance. The German model stimulated several countries to follow, especially Denmark between 1891 and 1998 and Belgium between 1894 and 1903; among the followers were also Switzerland and Sweden. Not at least the UK joined, which was already the pioneer of industrialization, developing social laws since 1906 and introducing its own Beveridge welfare state reforms after 1945 (Bahle et al. 2010).

All in all the welfare state concept was spreading in different forms through European nations; sometimes, it was well developed and later denominated the "social-democratic" type of welfare state; sometimes, it remained uncomplete and is now called a "rudimentary" type of welfare state. In other cases, the conservative type and the liberal type of welfare state came into existence. The welfare state was pushed through in long-during conflicts between the powerful societal forces of capital and labour. Often the welfare state was expanded in the countries; sometimes, trials for rolling back the welfare state came on schedule. But the welfare state was sustainably protected by many defenders (Atkinson 2001).

The claims of the concepts for welfare are not too far from the concepts of well-being (Holtmann 2018, p. 2ff). According to a classical concept, the welfare state was described as follows: "The essence of the welfare state is government protected minimum standards of income, nutrition, health assured to every citizen as a right, not as a charity" (Wilensky 1975, p. 1). Whereas in this concept the welfare state is concentrated on support of the poor, in recent definitions the modern welfare state is regarded as going beyond this goal and defined its task as "Well-Being for All" (Council of Europe 2008). The welfare goals of modern welfare state are no longer restricted to maintain minimum standards for poor minorities; moreover, they are related to the well-being of the whole population. The welfare state activities have nowadays a broad influence on the well-being for all which implies the risk that improving the lot of the disadvantaged is somewhat neglected.

In Europe, five types of welfare states are distinguished (Esping-Andersen 1990; Glatzer and Kohl 2017; Holtmann 2018, p. 50)[1]: social democratic, conservative, liberal, rudimentary and post-socialist.

Advocates of the **liberal** version of the welfare state believe in the superior efficiency of market production and distribution of rewards. Therefore, they do not see a necessity for political interventions in market mechanisms, but rather regard them as detrimental. For the same reason, they also want to restrict the public provision of goods and services to "pure" public goods (such as defence, police, courts) and to exclude those services which can also be provided by private markets.

---

[1] This subchapter and especially the types of welfare states are conceptualized by Jürgen Kohl in our common article (Glatzer and Kohl 2017), and they are similar designed in the international comparison by Holtmann (2018). The origin of this conceptualization is Esping-Anderson (1990).

Proponents of the **conservative–corporatist** welfare state do not share the unconditional belief of the liberals in the superiority of markets. On the one hand, they basically accept the capitalist market economy, but recognize the necessity to regulate markets, especially labour markets, in order to avoid negative consequences of capitalist production, above all exploitation of labour and mass poverty. On the other hand, they also recognize a role for the state to care for the subsistence of those parts of the population which is not integrated into the active labour force (the sick, the elderly, children, housewives).

Advocates of the **social-democratic** welfare state do not believe in the "*distributive justice*" of capitalist market economies (although they generally accept their "allocative efficiency"), but want (and feel legitimized) to correct the distributive results by political means in various ways. First, they put a high emphasis on social citizenship rights which in their interpretation means less inequality of living conditions among the citizens, not just the absence of poverty. Second, they put a high priority to the public provision of goods and services in order to make up for the deficiencies of private markets. Third, they recognize the necessity to regulate labour markets and thereby to limit the scope for inequality in the distribution of market income on the one hand and to secure high levels of employment on the other.

The **rudimentary** welfare state shares many of the characteristics of the conservative–corporatist model, but attributes a lesser role to the state. Public schemes for social protection and state-run social services are less developed. Instead—following the subsidiarity principle—more responsibility for people's well-being is assigned to families and kinship (as the smallest social communities) and to voluntary charitable organizations, above all those run by the churches.

The **post-socialist** welfare state, in contrast, shares certain features of the social-democratic model, in particular the concern for equality of living conditions and the preference for government intervention to achieve these results. More importantly, the countries classified as "post-socialist" are still characterized by the legacies of their past from the post-war period up to the 1990s.

There is broad agreement about the countries type of welfare state though sometimes features are overlapping. According to the study of Holtmann (2018, p. 50), the types of welfare states in Europe are the following: the social-democratic welfare state type is represented in its most typical form in the Nordic countries as Denmark, Finland, Sweden and outside the EU in Norway. The conservative type of the welfare state is most clearly realized in the Central European countries such as Austria, Belgium, France, Germany and Luxembourg. The liberal welfare state type is—as far as Europe is concerned—approximated by the UK and Ireland. Characteristics of the rudimentary welfare state—also called the family-oriented type due to the family's role in social support—are typically found in the Southern European countries such as Italy, Portugal, Spain and also Cyprus, Malta and Greece. Finally, there are the post-socialist countries in Central Eastern Europe like Bulgaria, Czech Republic, Hungary, Poland, Slovak Republic, Romania and Slovenia. In the North-East of Europe the Baltic states of Estonia, Latvia and Lithuania are classified under the label of the post-socialist regime type.[2]

The performance of the welfare state can find its expression in many fields. But there are three goal areas which are central, namely the goals of sustaining self-sufficiency, the reduction of poverty and the modification of inequality.

Sustaining self-sufficiency. "Self-sufficiency is promoted by ensuring active social and economic participation by people" (OECD 2009, p. 53). First of all, it is guaranteed by paid employment which provides the economic resources to enable people to live a life "self-sufficiently". People should be able to support themselves and their families from their earnings without contributions from others, in particular not from social transfers of the government. Only in case they are—temporarily or permanently—unable to earn their living by paid employment, the state is responsible to provide a sufficient substitute. Unwanted as well is especially the case of earnings from full employment that are not enough to guarantee a decent subsistence.

Employment rates are on the average the highest in the countries of the social-democratic regime type (see blue line in Fig. 7.3). All the countries belonging to this type have since some time shown employment rates between 73 and 82% of the adult population of 15–64 years, rates which have been reached less often in other countries. Conservative welfare states have not attained an employment rate of 80% and are sometimes below 70%. Central European countries following the conservative model of the state are performing less with respect to employment. The two countries of the liberal type are on similar levels as the conservative welfare states. Below the employment rate of all these countries are the post-socialist countries of Central and Eastern Europe. And the lowest rates of employment are attained in the rudimentary welfare states of Southern Europe. They mostly remain below the EU average of 71%, and they reach partly only employment rates of 60% and below (Fig. 9.1).

The main reason for the cross-national differences in employment rates lies in the different levels of the inclusion of women in the labour markets. The employment

---

[2]The quality of data of some smaller countries (for instance, the Baltic States, Malta and Cyprus) appears to be less reliable and has been excluded from this analysis.

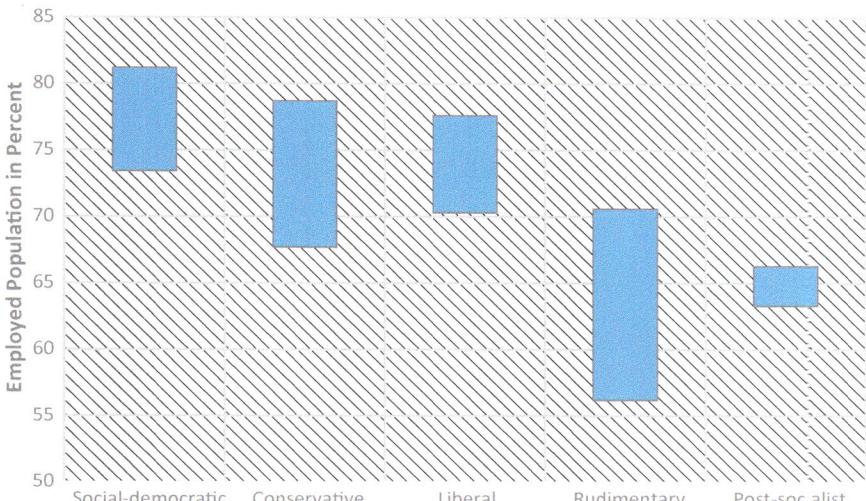

Fig. 9.1 Employment rates for persons aged 20 to 64 by types of welfare states in the European Union 2016. *Reading example* The employment rates of social-democratic welfare states have values between 73 and 82% and of the conservative welfare states between 67 and 78%. *Source* Eurostat—statistics explained: employment statistics (own construction)

rates of men are more on a similar level and show a slightly decreasing trend over time. But the labour force participation rates of women differ sharply although they have been rising in almost all European countries over the last decades, with certain time lags. In the Scandinavian countries, employment rates of men and women are almost the same, especially among the younger cohorts. But in almost all other European countries, there is a marked difference between male and female employment rates of sometimes more than 10% points. Surprisingly, female employment rates are fairly low in post-socialist countries, despite the ideological claims of gender equality under their former regimes (Fig. 9.2).

Employment made people in European countries more satisfied with their life, and unemployment, especially if it was for a longer time, reduced their satisfaction with life. The sometimes told story that the unemployed enjoy a life without working is almost wrong. If people are without employment, then their life satisfaction is low. And life satisfaction is also much lower for the retired people and the so-called homemakers than for the employed. Employment contributes to life satisfaction. Only students are the exception, who enjoy their life most.

Unemployment is statistically the other side of employment: indicating the *lack* of economic participation and a *loss of income*. There are numerous studies which show severe social and psychological consequences of unemployment, especially in the case of long-term unemployment. The comparison of unemployment rates across

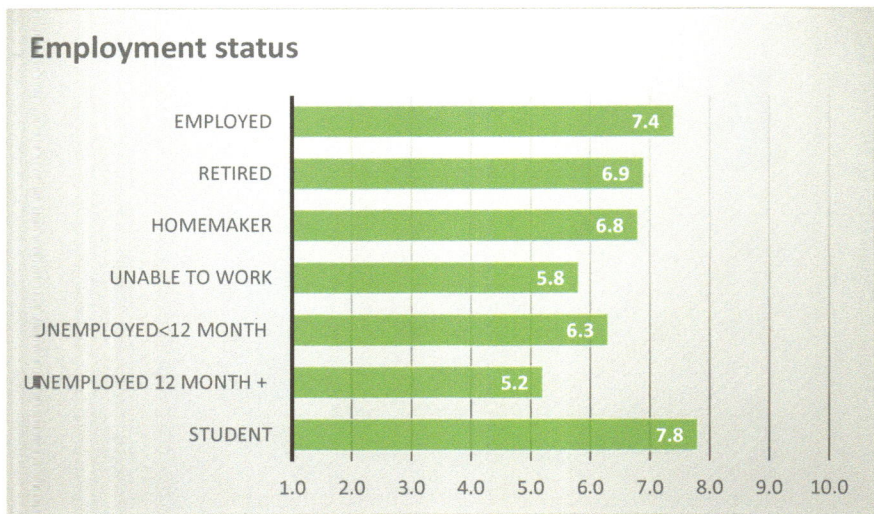

Fig. 9.2 Life satisfaction by employment status in the EU 2016. *Note* Life satisfaction is measured on the 10-point scale from 1 to 10. *Source* Eurofound (2017), European Quality of Life Survey (2016) p. 16

European countries shows a similar pattern as for employment rates.[3] With respect to the different types of welfare states, unemployment rates are the smallest in favour of the social-democratic welfare states.

People at Risk of Poverty. Preventing poverty is of high priority in the European Union political affairs[4] (Ott and Wagner 1997, p. 1), and it is clear in the awareness of social–political scientists, who postulate strongly that poverty rates should be reduced (Atkinson 2001). Among the risk-of-poverty rates, the poverty measurement of Eurostat is well recognized which speaks of a "risk of poverty" and not substantially of "poverty". In the social-democratic welfare states, the risk-of-poverty rates are the lowest. In the conservative and the liberal welfare regimes, rates are below 10%, whereas the countries with a rudimentary and post-socialist welfare states suffer from risk-of-poverty rates often far above 10%. The post-socialist welfare states of the East do not attain the same high risk-of-poverty rates of the rudimentary welfare states of Western Europe (Fig. 9.3).

---

[3]Though there is a certain complementarity between employment and unemployment, there are also inconsistencies; while there is a considerable gender gap with regard to the level of employment—there is virtually no such gender gap with regard to unemployment.

[4]At risk of poverty or social exclusion, abbreviated as AROPE, refers to the situation of people either at risk of poverty or severely materially deprived or living in a household with a very low work intensity. This is the headline indicator for monitoring the EU 2020 strategy poverty target.

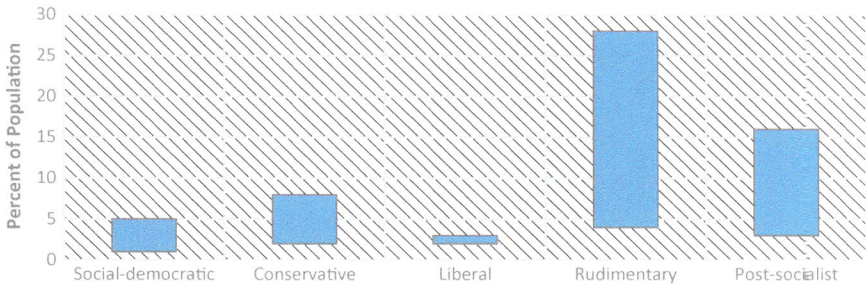

Fig. 9.3 At-risk-of-poverty rates by type of welfare state in EU Member States 2016. *Note* The at-risk-of-poverty rate is the share of people with an equivalized disposable income below the at-risk-of-poverty threshold which is set at 60% of the national median equivalized disposable income after social transfers (own construction). *Reading example* Social-democratic welfare states show a risk-of-poverty rate between 1 and 5%, post-socialist welfare states between 3 and 16% depending on one of the states. *Source* http://ec.europa.eu/eurostat/statisticsexplained/index.phGlossary:At_risk_of_poverty_or_social

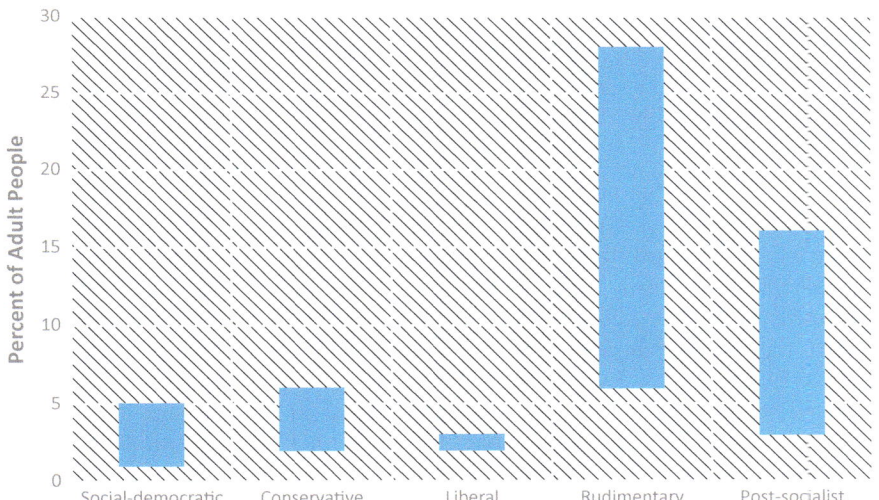

Fig. 9.4 People who have strong difficulties to make ends meet by type of welfare state in EU Member States 2016. *Source* Eurofound (2018), European Quality of Life Survey 2016 (data received by email from Eurofound/Dublin, own construction)

In the time course of the last two decades, the risk of poverty has been rising in most European countries, but relatively more in those countries where poverty rates have initially been low. On the other hand, poverty has even gone down in some countries with initially high poverty rates (Fig. 9.4).

Strong difficulties to make ends meet can be regarded as an expression of the subjective feeling of poverty. This subjective perception of poverty behaves parallel

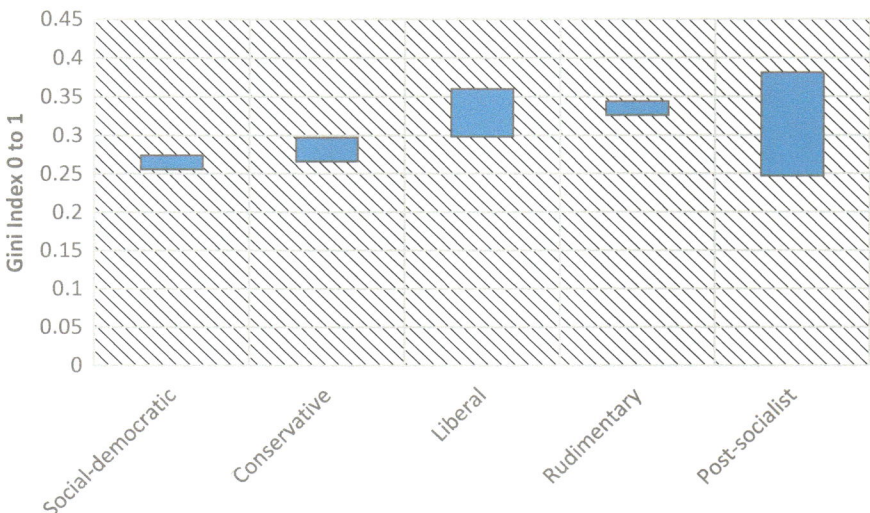

Fig. 9.5 Income inequality measured by Gini index in different types of European welfare states 2016. *Note* The Gini index for the disposable equivalized income runs from 0 to 1 and indicates perfect equality of income with 0 and perfect inequality with 1. Higher values indicate higher inequality of the income distribution (own construction). *Source* Eurostat, Data Explorer, 31 August 2018

to the objective amount of poverty measured according to poverty borders of experts. People in social-democratic welfare states report the lowest difficulties to make ends meet. People in the conservative and the liberal welfare states are not much worse. The most difficulties exist according to the statements of the people in the rudimentary welfare states. Rather high difficulties to make ends meet are also present in post-socialist welfare states. The success of the social-democratic welfare states will be expected because they are known for their better-off in employment. People react finally with their subjective perception according to their objective conditions.

Modifying Income Inequality. The existing amount of economic inequality is often criticized, and it has its influence on well-being (Boehnke and Kohler 2010). The optimistic expectation is that "less inequality benefits all" (OECD 2015). The welfare states organize redistribution from the primary market distribution of the production factors into a secondary distribution of disposable income in the private households. This is always a significant contribution to more income equality. The disposable inequality is usually measured with the Gini index for the equivalized disposable income (Fig. 9.5).

Concerning the inequality of disposable income, there is a fairly clear rank order of regime types, as suggested by welfare state regime theory: countries following the social-democratic model show the lowest inequality, the conservative welfare states show a higher inequality, and the countries of the liberal cluster are again higher with their income inequality. The rudimentary welfare states are on similar levels

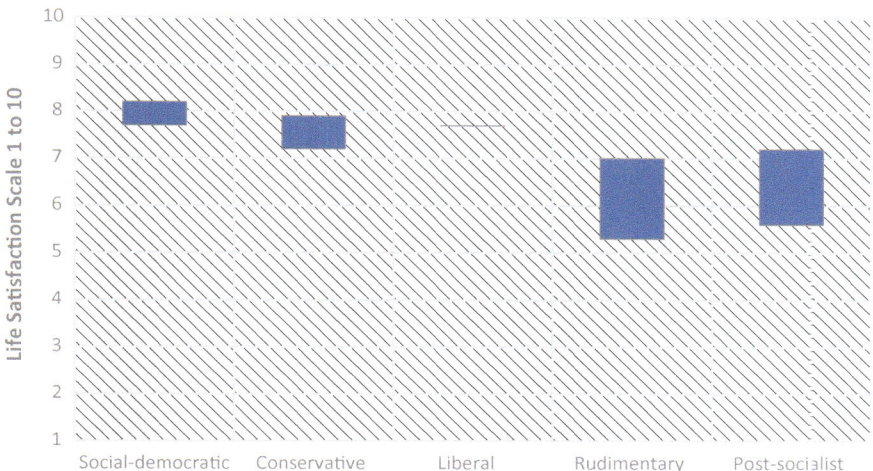

Fig. 9.6 Satisfaction with life according to the type of welfare state in EU Member States 2016. *Source* Eurofound (2018), European Quality of Life Survey 2016 (data received by email from Eurofound/Dublin, own construction)

with the liberal welfare states. The post-socialist countries of Central and Eastern Europe are characterized by surprisingly low income inequality. It is suggested that this is most likely due to low inequality in the primary income distribution—as part of their socialist heritage—rather than to redistributive activities of their current welfare states. Extreme income inequality remains a source of social conflicts in and between European countries (Stiglitz 2012) and a threat for their cohesion.

Satisfaction with life according to the type of welfare state. The three indicators used above for the performance of the welfare states are usually classified as "objective" indicators which tell how scientific experts evaluate according to their knowledge the state of affairs. How people see personally their living conditions is another question usually measured by the satisfaction of people. The measure of life satisfaction as it is implemented often in national, international and global survey can be regarded as a summary indicator of the *subjective state of the nation*, which varies according to the types of welfare states (Fig. 9.6).

Life satisfaction in Europe is according to the results of European and international surveys obviously correlated with the type of welfare state in various countries (Glatzer and Kohl 2017, p. 446). In the Eurostat Quality of Life survey of the year 2016, the highest average life satisfaction is reported for citizens in the social-democratic welfare states in the range from 7.8 to 8.2. Somewhat lower but not too much is the average life satisfaction in the conservative and the liberal welfare states. People in rudimentary welfare states attain much lower levels of life satisfaction in the range from 5.6 to 7.1. Some of the post-socialist states are on a deeper level, but some are better than the rudimentary welfare states.

There is less doubt that the institutional arrangements of the different types of welfare states are influencing individual well-being significantly, in particular by supporting self-sufficiency, by reducing poverty and by modifying income distribution.

The highest satisfaction with life in Europe is attained in the case of Norway, which is situated outside the European Union. In Norway, people have a unique constellation of prosperity and welfare which is due to a combination of the wealth from oil reservoirs in the North Sea together with the model of a social-democratic welfare state. It is rather convincing that a combination of high prosperity and social-democratic welfare leads to the highest fulfilment of Europeans' well-being. But this optimal constellation is not attainable for all.

References

Atkinson, T. (2001). *The economic consequences of rolling back the welfare state*. Cambridge, Massachusetts, London: The MIT Press.

Bahle, T., Kohl, J., & Wendt, C. (2010). Welfare state. In S. Immerfall & G. Therborn (Eds.), *Handbook of European Societies. Social Transformations in the 21st Century* (pp. 571–628). New York, NY, Dordrecht, London: Springer.

Boehnke, P., & Kohler, U. (2010). Well-Being and Inequality. In C. Immerfall & G. Therborn (Eds.), *Handbook of European Societies. Social Transformations in the 21st Century* (pp. 629–666). New York, Dordrecht, London, Heidelberg: Springer.

Briggs, A. (2000). The welfare state in historical perspective. In C. Pierson, & F. Castles (Eds.), *The Welfare State Reader* (pp. 11–17). Oxford: Blackwell Publishers.

Council of Europe. (2008). *Well-being for all: Concepts and tools for social cohesion*. Strasbourg: Council of Europe Publishing.

Esping-Anderson, G. (1990). *The three worlds of welfare capitalism*. Princeton, New York: Princeton University Press.

Eurofound. (2017). *European Quality of Life Survey 2016. Quality of life, Quality of public services, and Quality of society*. Luxembourg: Publications Office of the European Union.

Glatzer, W., & Kohl, J. (2017). The History of Well-being in Europe. In R. J. Estes & M. J. Sirgy (Eds.), *The Pursuit of Human well-being* (pp. 409–452). Switzerland: Springer.

Hollmann, D. (2018). *43 Country case studies on the performance of politics, economy and society*. Aachen: Shaker Verlag.

OECD. (2009). *Society at a glance 2009*. OECD Social Indicators: OECD-Publishing.

OECD. (2015). *In it together—why less inequality benefits all*. Paris: OECD-Publishing.

Ott, N., & Wagner, G. (1997). *Income inequality and poverty in Eastern and Western Europe*. Heidelberg: Physica Verlag.

Stiglitz, J. (2012). *The price of inequality: How today's divided society endangers our future*. New York London: W.W. Norton & Company.

Wilensky, H. (1975). *The welfare state and equality*. Berkeley, Los Angeles, London: University of California Press.

Chapter 10
Variety and Inequality of Well-Being

Abstract Inequality inside and between societies is a topic that attracts a lot of critical attention from public and science. The diagnosis if a society is characterized by inequality or heterogeneity or by variety or diversity is not easy to meet. The basic questions are which context has high and which one has low inequality scores and what are the causes and what are the social consequences, for example social tensions. Each society is constituted from different population groups. There are always big groups of the population who are unequal according to gender, age, education, income and migration. The ranking of these groups according to their life satisfaction gives an impression of the subjective differentiation of the population. An interesting point is also if individuals include in their well-being different levels of satisfaction. In Europe, satisfaction with the own family is high and satisfaction with standard of living is relatively low. This is called the horizontal disparity of individuals' satisfaction. Each of people is confronted with the question how much variety and inequality should be accepted for living just and fair together.

Vertical Disparities of Satisfaction with Life. Each population is stratified and contains disparities and sometimes conflict lines. Main population groups are presented in the following table for the European Union with respect to gender, age categories, education, income and migrants (Eurofound 2017, Ahrend et al. 2015). Two extraordinary deficit groups with respect to life satisfaction are added, namely unemployed and sick, respectively, handicapped people. Life satisfaction constitutes a stratification of its own and varies significantly with social structural variables.

Figure 10.1 gives a comprehensive description of the life satisfaction of social structural groups of the population of all the European countries which shows at one view the difference between the population categories. The overall picture is the following population groups: at the top of high life satisfaction in European societies are the people with tertiary education, the age category 18–24 years, and the people within the highest income quartile. At the bottom of life satisfaction are two categories of people. These are the people, who are long-term unemployed and people with health restrictions, who are sick or handicapped. Other groups are in between these top-satisfied and low-satisfied people.

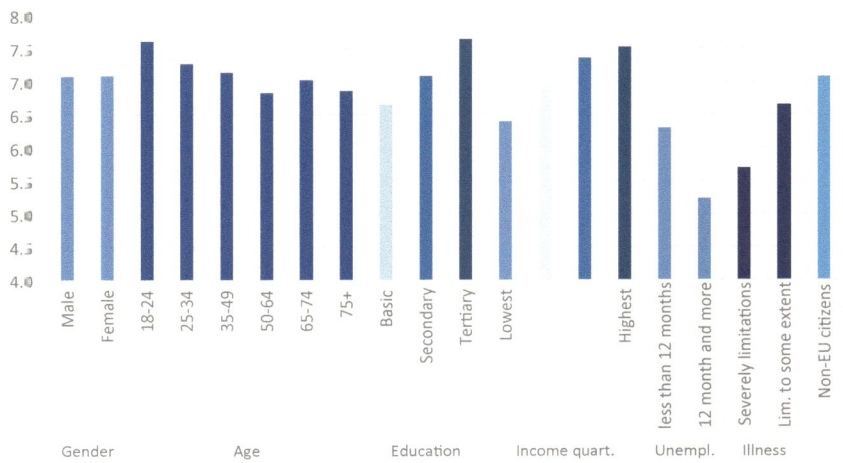

Fig. 10.1 Life satisfaction for socio-structural population groups in the European Union 2016. *Note* Income quart. = Income quartile; Unempl. = Unemployed. *Source* Euro found (2017). European Quality of Life Survey 2016. p. 16

Gender. The gender difference of well-being in Europe is complex and partially contradictory. All things considered, men and women in Europe express the same life satisfaction of 7.1 on the ten-point scale (European Union 2017). This is in some contrast to the view that usually women's life situation is diagnosed as disadvantageous, and therefore, one would expect that their subjective well-being is below men's life satisfaction (Eckermann 2017, pp. 609–637). This is not the case for Europe as a whole but varies in the European countries; sometimes, women are more satisfied than men, and sometimes, men are more satisfied than women. Significantly more satisfied men than women are found in Hungary, Slovenia and Italy. More satisfied women than men are present in Finland, Ireland and Denmark. The gender disparity has developed in the countries very differently. A number of countries have reached a satisfaction balance between the sexes, for example Germany, Great Britain, Switzerland, Sweden, Spain, Netherland and Luxembourg. As we have to attribute these outcomes, at least partially, to the women's movement in Europe, then the movement was not equally successful in the different countries of Europe (Eckermann 2017).

Of additional relevance for the gender balance is that men and women have different sources of satisfaction. If quality of life is regarded in terms of an affect balance, then it comes out that women's experience is different from men's life experience (Bradburn 2015). The "affect balance scale", which shows different scores for men and women in European countries, shows for women report less positive affect than for men (OECD 2015, p. 274). In most European countries, the affect balance score is higher for men which means there are more positive emotional events for men during a day. Only in very few countries women are better off in their affect balance than men, namely in Sweden and Finland. Women's emancipation is a rather differentiated task. And up to now a more amenable life for women took only place in the north of Europe.

Age. For each individual, ageing is a non-escapable process, and probably, satisfaction varies with the life course of the individuals. It is different for societies who can grow older or younger, but most European societies are exposed to the risk to grow older. We do not know very much about how satisfaction is related to the life course of individuals because measurement in Europe is mainly a comparison of age groups. In a cross-sectional comparison of age groups, the differences in satisfaction show for Europe as a whole the following pattern: highest satisfaction has the youngest age group from 15 to 25. Lowest satisfaction can be found in the oldest age group above 75. In between the life satisfaction is step for step lower with higher age groups. But the exception is the age group between 65 and 75. They are below the group which is younger and above the age group which is older.

In Europe, the population is usually divided into three large age groups. The size of these groups is characterized by an increase in the population share of the older ones and a decrease in the number of younger people (Eurofound 2017, p. 15).

More important is that the satisfaction with life is a very flexible point. Each country shows its special step pattern. In some countries, life satisfaction seems to be on the same level in the three age groups which is an equality pattern (e.g. Denmark, Austria et al.). In other countries, the loss of satisfaction with life happens between the younger and the middle age groups and is compensated for the older ones (e.g. the Netherlands, Germany et al.). The satisfaction level of the younger ones is in their countries not on the lowest level, but in country comparisons, it is demonstrated that in countries such as Italy, Bulgaria and Greece it is nevertheless dramatically low.

The balance of satisfaction levels between age groups is a political task. It seems that there are some age differences of well-being in Europe, but they are not severe enough to constitute a significant source for conflicts.

Education. Education has spread in the last centuries successfully in Western and Eastern Europe. In both areas is the population, which has attained at least basic education, close to 100% and the average years of education are 11–12 years (van Zanden 2014, p. 94). Education brings many benefits, and this goes far beyond better position in economy and society far into subjective well-being (European Union 2015). Education is a bridge to higher life satisfaction. People with low educational degrees show much less life satisfaction than people with secondary and tertiary degrees (Euro found 2017, p. 16). Educational degrees seem to create important satisfaction gaps in different dimensions of society. Among EU countries, Portugal, Spain, Slovenia and Hungary have particular large gaps between people with and people without tertiary education. In contrast, Ireland, Sweden, Denmark and Norway have small education-related gaps (OECD 2016, p. 171). Poor countries tend to develop higher-education-related satisfaction gaps than countries with higher per capita income.

As far as we see, the satisfaction benefits of higher educational degrees will diminish in the future, when it goes on that more and more people attain the higher degrees. Education will loose of its capacity to produce individual satisfaction.

Income. It is usually empirical evident that higher-income strata—as the higher income quartiles in Fig. 10.1—have higher life satisfaction scores than lower-income strata. This is not astonishing because money opens the way to most goods of the world. No wonder that the highest-income strata attain highest life satisfaction. Astonishing was the paradox postulated by Easterlin (2015) about the relationship between economic growth and happiness with life in worldwide perspective including European countries. Growing income is in the time course not accompanied by growing satisfaction with life. "The evidence also indicates that the frequently cited cross-section relation of happiness to income is not reproduced in time series, where the long term relation tends to be nil" (Easterlin 2015, p. 297). A reason may be that income is used for consumption and the spending of income for consumption does not contribute always to well-being: "The literature shows that growth in consumption is not positively related with increases in well-being" (Guillen-Royo and Langford-Wilhite 2015, p 312).

The satisfaction difference between high- and low-income strata is relatively high, and it is often stated that it challenges social cohesion. In particular, the huge discrepancy between highest and lowest incomes, which arises due to the potentials of globalization, may be perceived as a threat.

Minorities and Migration. Europe is part of a global migration system, and it has no chance to escape its challenges (Bös 2007). "Increasingly, with globalization, the people of the world are on the move, and most of these migrants are seeking a happier life" (Helliwell et al. 2018, Chap. 1). There is no imagination that globalization could happen without an increase in migration. "There are large gaps in happiness between countries and these will continue to create major pressures to migrate" (Helliwell et al. 2018, Chap. 1). The main migration problem of today is a stream of immigrants coming from the north of Africa and the near east to Europe. The goal of migrants to attain at higher satisfaction is not attained also not on the long run. Migrants remain above their home satisfaction level but below their host-country satisfaction level. In this case Fig. 10.1 shows that life satisfaction of non-EU citizen is under proportional compared with EU-citizen.

People who try to overcome the protected borders of Europe across the Mediterranean Sea shipwreck frequently. The deaths at Europe's southern border bring an unsolvable challenge to the Europeans who intend to control and distribute the migrant streams in the European countries. The new migrants enlarge the group of older migrants, who often after two or three generations are only partially integrated in their host country. The early migrants from several decades and centuries ago are nearly not distinguishable—only by their names—from the native population, e.g. in Germany the Sorbs in the Lusatia, the Huguenots in Prussian territories and the Polish workers in the coal and steel area of the "Ruhrgebiet". In the long run time works for integration but generations of migrants develop their own habits of integration and segregation.

Minorities are defined as groups of ethnic and linguistic homogeneity within a national population, and preferably, they are object to prejudice and also physical attacks. The number of ethnic minorities in the single European countries is estimated; rather, different and total estimations are given between 54 and 300 million or according to another guess 14% of European population.[1] Examples for ethnic minorities in Europe are manifold: Jews, Sinti and Roma, Sorbs, Basks. Some peoples are majority in one country and minority in another one as the Danes in Germany. The minorities result mostly from migration between different parts of Europe, and this has a millennial history and happened in big waves. It still exercises a lot of pressure in contemporary Europe.

The general attitude towards migrants has been studied by an indirect question: "people think that the city or area where they live is a good place to live for immigrants?" (OECD 2014, p. 137). The results, which may have changed somewhat in recent times, show that there is a strong North–South cleavage with respect to the definition of good societies for migrants: the inhabitants of 90% of Iceland, Norway and Sweden define their countries as good living places for migrants. On the other hand, less than 50% of the adult population of Poland, Estonia and Greece do not see their country as a good place for migrants. There may be different reasons for this, like a poor economic situation of the native population or an in-group attitude which is hostile towards foreigners. By regarding areas with smaller and higher shares of migrants, one can learn that the percentage of migrants is not important in regard to the question how friendly or hostile they are perceived. The migration problem will remain one of the major conflict potential as long as the well-being gap and the resulting tension between Europe and North Africa are not reduced.

The minorities receive special attention as from the Council of Europe who declared in 1995 the Framework Convention for the Protection of National Minorities. Our current state of knowledge does not allow to make a general statement about their well-being in Europe. In Table 18 is documented that migrants from non-EU countries have a lower but not very low life satisfaction. This is an usual result from other surveys too that migrants have a higher life satisfaction than in their home country but a lower one than the native population. As far as we know, the integration needs several generations to be successful.

Unemployment. Since the early investigation of the effects of unemployment during the World Economic Crisis, the people in Europe know about the fatal effects of losing or not having a job (Jahoda et al. 1933). That the unemployed are living with fun on the costs of the employed people is a story far away from the negative psychosocial consequences of unemployment. As unemployment differs extremely between European countries the consequences are different amounts of well-being for people and societies. The extreme values of the unemployment rate exist in 2018 between the Southern Europe and the Continental Europe.[2] Destruction of well-

---

[1] (en.wikipedia.org/wiki/Ethnic_groups_in_Europe).

[2] https://www.statista.com/statistics/268830/unemployment-rate-in-eu-countries/. In June 2018, the figures are for Greece (20.2%), Spain (15.2%) and Italy (10.9%) on the negative side and for Czech Republic (2.4%) and Germany (3.4%) on the positive side.

being by unemployment can be very hard, and it differs according to the length of unemployment. To be unemployed more than a year is accompanied by the lowest average life satisfaction which exists in Europe (Fig. 10.1). As economists state that a certain degree of unemployment is unavoidable, it should be the task of state and society to meliorate unemployment and its consequences.

Health and Sickness. It belongs to the great positive feature of mankind that many people live long and feel healthy. The last health measurement in the EU countries in 2013 showed that 91% perceived their health as positive—among them 68% as good and very good, 23% as fair. On the other side there are 9% perceiving the own health as bad or very bad (European Union 2015, p. 115). The subjective feeling about the own health may be not accurate, but the positive feeling about the own health is a necessary contribution to the own well-being. If there are severe health limitations or health limitations to some extent, then life satisfaction goes significantly down (Fig. 10.1). Illness implies in general a certain reduction of life satisfaction, and it has a lot of further impacts on well-being as the limitation of activities.

Life in Europe is accompanied by a steady increase in people in higher age groups who describe their health as bad and very bad[3] (European Union 2015, p. 113). The increase in illness with age is in principle unavoidable, but a challenge is the huge differences between the countries. The percentage of adults reporting a long-standing illness or health problem varies in European countries from Ireland with 81% people in good health to Croatia 42% good health (European Union 2015, p. 113). That there exists a strong potential for country-specific deficits of life satisfaction through illness and unemployment defines a task for society to help the needy ones (Fig. 7.1).

A successful minimizing of unemployment and an empathic controlling of illness could make a significant contribution to the life satisfaction of most European people.

Horizontal Disparities of Well-Being. The topic of horizontal disparities has been raised in studies some decades ago. It is related to the problem of higher and lower levels which the same people attain in different life domains. If for example a low level of the quality of accommodation is accompanied by a high level of entertainment, this may create a tension for the household. It would make sense for the household members to increase satisfaction with accommodation and to invest less into entertainment. In the early studies, there were concentric circles representing different levels of the provision with certain goods. It was stated that some goods had a higher provisional degree and others a lower one. This view can be transferred to the satisfaction with "goods". According to theoretical expectations, it would make sense that people try to attain a similar level of satisfaction in all life domains. But empirical studies of satisfaction levels show that this is not the case in Europe: European responses indicate hierarchical ladders of satisfaction in which family life is at the top of the satisfaction ladder and standard of living is much lower. In between

---

[3]Whereas in the age group 16–24 the percentage of people who report bad or very bad health is 1.4%, the percentage for the 75+ age group is 29.7% with a regular increase in between (European Union 2015, p. 117).

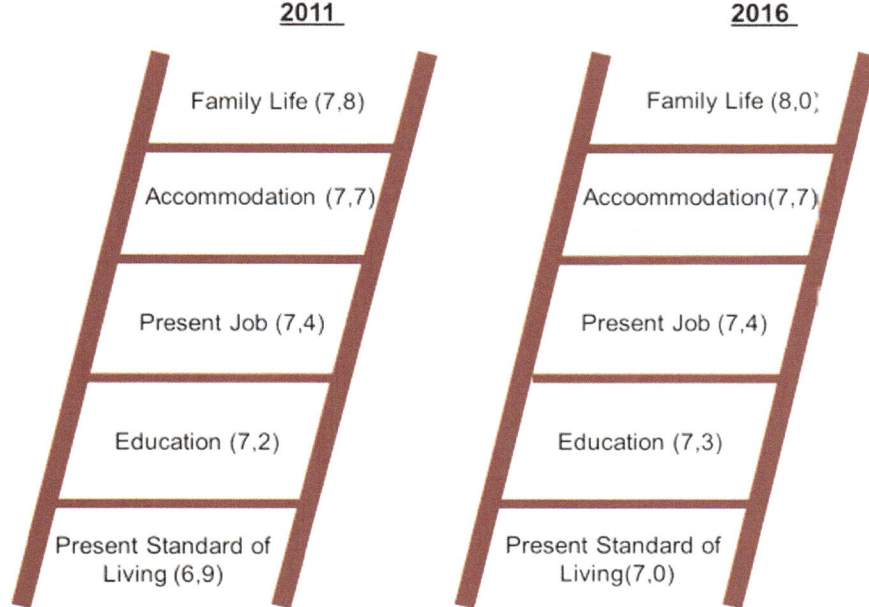

Fig. 10.2 Average satisfaction for selected life domains in the European Union (28) in the years 2011 and 2016. *Note* satisfaction scales from 1 to 10. Additional domains were investigated in 2016: satisfaction with the way democracy works in [country] (5.2) Satisfaction with the present state of the economy in [country] (4.9). *Source* European Union (2017), European Quality of Life Surveys 2011 and 2016

are accommodation, job and education—in this order (Fig. 10.2).[4] According to these results, European ways of living look somewhat post-material.

In another European survey in 2013, we find a similar picture: at the top of the satisfaction ladder "satisfaction with personal relationships" and at the bottom the "satisfaction with the financial situation of the household" (European Union 2015, p. 155, p. 20).[5] According to scientific expectations, the domain of "social relations" is more satisfying in Europe than the domain "financial situation". Most impressive is the stable rank order between 2011 and 2016 and also in 2013. Though Europe was developing in the last centuries to a high level of prosperity, it was not attaining the same high satisfaction level for their standard of living as they attain for their family life and their personal relations.[6]

The individuals are surrounded by satisfaction levels which show a clear order. All the satisfaction ladders are confirming this effect. One could suppose that the

[4]The actual scarcity of adequate accommodations, to which Europe is exposed nowadays, is a rather new phenomenon and will surely appear as a result in the future surveys.

[5]The values for the satisfaction with housing are 2013 within the two extremes.

[6]In the Eurofound Quality of Life Survey of 2013, different terms are used with personal relations on the top and financial situation on the bottom of the satisfaction scale.

needs of people in material respect are more difficult to satisfy than with respect to their social relations. It seems as if Europeans have reached the age of post-materialism and invest more energy in the satisfaction of immaterial needs than in material goods. Also very important is that family life or personal relations; if they are boring, they can be finished by separation and divorce. If material living conditions are dissatisfying, it is more difficult to escape. It remains a problem for European people that they are leading in the world's material affluence, but people do not attain the same satisfaction as in immaterial life domains.

There are further topics which show, with respect to their satisfaction level, a lower level than the material conditions. In 2016, these levels were the satisfaction with the way democracy works (5.2) and the satisfaction with the development of the national economy (4.9). These relatively low satisfaction values express that European people are in most cases more critical towards their collective circumstances than towards their private circumstances. Theoretically, it seems to be easier to be dissatisfied with collective phenomena than with private conditions (Glatzer 2008). A reason may be that the responsibility for private conditions is individual and the responsibility or collective phenomena is shared among many people.

References

Ahrendt, D., Dubois, H., & Mezger, E. (2015). An overview of quality of life and well-being in Europe. In W. Glatzer, L. Camfield, V. Moller, & M. Roja (Eds.), *Global Handbook of Quality of Life*. Dordrecht: Springer.

Bös M. (2007). Ethnizität und Grenzen in Europa. In P. Deger & R. Hettlage (Eds.), Europäischer Raum und Grenzen. Probleme der Räumlichkeit und Identitätsbildung in einem vereinten Europa. Wiesbaden: VS-Verlag.

Bradburn, N. M. (2015). The affect balance scale: Subjective approaches. In W. Glatzer, L. Camfield, V Moller, & M. Roja (Eds.), *Global Handbook of Quality of Life*. Dordrecht: Springer.

Easterlin, R. A. (2015). Happiness and economic growth—the evidence. In W. Glatzer, L. Camfield, V Moller, & M. Roja (Eds.), *Global Handbook of Quality of Life* (pp. 283–299). Doordrecht: Springer.

Eckerman E. (2017). The History of Well-being and the Global Progress of Women. In R. Estes, & J. Sargy, J (Eds.), *The Pursuit of Human Well-Being*. Switzerland: Springer International Publishing.

European Union. (2015). *Quality of life—facts and views*. Luxembourg: Eurostat, Statistical Books.

European Union. (2017). *European Quality of Life Survey 2016. Quality of life, Quality of public services, and Qualty of society*. Luxembourg: Publications Office of the European Union.

Glatzer, W. (2008). Well-being: Perception and Measurement. In Council of Europe (Ed.), *Well-being for all: Concepts and Tools for Social Cohesion* (pp. 99–118). Strasbourg: Council of Europe Publishing.

Guillen-Royo, M., & Langford-Wilhite, H. (2015). Wellbeing and sustainable consumption. In W. Glatzer, L. Camfield, V. Moller, & M. Rojas (Eds.), *2015* (pp. 301–316). Springer, Dordrecht: Global Handbook of Quality of Life.

Helliwell, J., Layard, R., & Sachs, J. (2018). *World Happiness Report 2018*. New York: Sustainable Development Solutions Network.

Jahoda M., Lazarsfeld P. F., & Zeisel H. (1960/1933): Die Arbeitslosen von Marienthal. Verlag für Demoskopie: Allensbach und Bonn.

OECD. (2014). *Society at a Glance 2014. OECD Social Indicators*. Paris: OECD Publishing.

OECD. (2015). *How's Life. Measuring Well-being*. OECD Publishing.

OECD. (2016). *OECD-Factbook 2015–2016. Economic, Environmental and Social Statistics*. Paris: OECD Publishing.

Van Zanden, J., et al. (eds.) (2014). How Was Life? Global Well-being since 1820. OECD Publishing.

Chapter 11
Well-Being in Everyday Life

Abstract Some dimensions of everyday life in Europe, which are diminishing the well-being of people, will now be regarded. Living alone in a one person-household, is in the European average accompanied by a lower well-being than it exists for couples or multi-person households. A moderate problem, which leads to some deficits in well-being, is missing social support in case of need and emergency that Europeans don't feel often "anxious at a night walk" is a criterion for a certain safety and security. That relationships between people need to be grounded on trust is a challenge for a good society but it is scarce in European societies. These everyday dimensions are always seen from the eyes of the people itself. Experts have diagnosed that in each EU Member States deficits of social justice exist and that the discrepancies between the countries are rather big.

Ways of life are characterized by social contacts and relations, which are fundamental for human existence. Of special importance is the primary group which constitutes the private household respectively its living arrangements of individuals. The private household is in the first line responsible for the social contacts of the people living together. Social contacts are a prerequisite for social support which can help to overcome difficult situations of individual needs and emergency. People can hardly live without a feeling of security which is an indicator for the trust that they are not always exposed to threats for their property and their life. Another basic dimension is trust among people and to institutions. The danger in case of a loss of trust can be that life is growing difficult and will be full of disappointments. Finally, a general measure for a good society is justice, which is relevant in many dimensions of society. This list is selective, but these dimensions were included in European surveys and indicators to show their characteristics.

Living arrangements. Human needs for social contacts, social bonds and social relations will be satisfied by people mostly inside their own home or household. There is a significant gap of life satisfaction between one and multi-person households. Living arrangements which consist of one person (33.6% within EU28/2017) constitute a context, which never contains in the average the life satisfaction of couples and multi-person households. Households which consist of one adult and a child

© The Author(s), under exclusive licence to Springer Nature Switzerland AG 2019   67
W. Glatzer, *History and Politics of Well-Being in Europe*, SpringerBriefs in Well-Being
and Quality of Life Research, https://doi.org/10.1007/978-3-030-05048-1_11

or more children (additional 4.3%) are also low with respect to their life satisfaction. There is nearly no dissatisfaction difference between the single-households and the households which consist of one adult and one or more children.

Living together as a married couple is obviously preferred in Europe may it be with children (24.9% in the EU average) or without children (20.0% in EU average). A variety of multi-person households exist aside (17.2%) having a life satisfaction level in between. Living alone is the highest in Sweden (51.4%), Europe and the lowest in Malta (13.1%) and Portugal (16.8%). More traditional societies are still resisting but the trend goes into the direction of the Swedish model.

Living single with the risk of social isolation is often a patchy solution. Nevertheless, living alone is the type of household which is since many years increasing over-proportional in Europe. It is often a compulsory solution which is taken on frequently by widowed, divorced or separated people. Also, there are growing numbers of ' singles", who met their decision autonomously to live without a partner. Both factors together contribute in all European countries to an increasing number of people living alone and at the same time a decreasing number of people living together, and this creates a challenge which affects differently the European societies (OECD 2014, p. 93).

According to our societal knowledge, "Living Alone" is on the march forward in Europe; the impression is that it is following the Swedish model. The assumption is that this process of singularization will contribute to diminish well-being in Europe.

Social contacts. As everybody knows social contacts can happen with varying frequency inside and outside the own family and the own household. On this background in European surveys, the frequency of social contacts with friends and with relatives is investigated. In EU countries, social contacts with friends and with relatives are normally high. The question in the Europe-wide surveys some years ago in 2006 was how often somebody meets friends and relatives at least once a week during a usual year.

A low frequency of social contacts with friends existed in Poland, France, Hungary and Czech Republic, relatively intensive social contacts with friends exist in Greece, Portugal and the Netherlands (OECD 2011, p. 175). As in other cases, there is a broad middle field between these extremes of social contacts with friends.

In regard to social contacts with relatives, there are also rather big differences. Social contacts with relatives are most often in Greece, Portugal and Belgium, whereas these contacts are low in Poland, Estonia and Denmark. "Countries where people socialize frequently with family members also tend to be those where people socialize more frequently with friends" (OECD 2011, p. 175). Presumedly, there are different social contact cultures in European countries which depend on the multiple historic experiences in each country.

Social support. Giving and receiving social support is essential for overcoming various problems, which accompany human life. Social support can be measured with the use of different questions. One example is the question if somebody is "not having anyone to rely on in case of need" which was included in the Eurostat survey 2013. The result for the European Union seems in the average with the value of 7% for having nobody in the case of need acceptable, but some countries show much higher deficits (Fig. 11.1). Some countries as Greece, Luxembourg and Italy are above 10% without social support, whereas Slovakia, Finland and Hungary have a very low deficit of about 2% (EU 2015, p. 152). There is a broad middle field in European society where the availability of social support is above 90%.

An overview about distortions in the dimensions of every well-being is given by the following table (Fig. 11.2).

Some years ago in an OECD survey, the percentage of people was counted who "have relatives or friends they can count on for help in times of need" (OECD 2011, p. 174). Also in this earlier survey was the result that social support is no scarce resource in the average. Already the weak countries Portugal, Estonia and Italy have

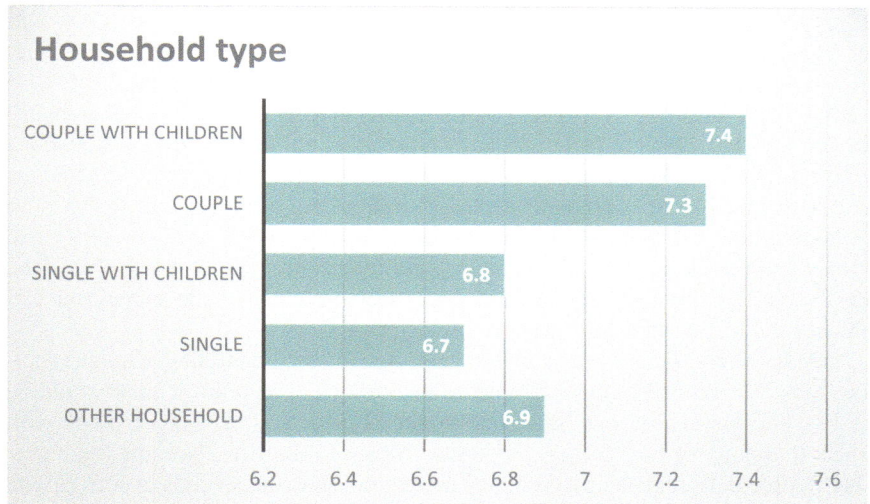

Fig. 11.1 Life satisfaction according to living arrangement in the European Union in the year 2016. *Note* Life satisfaction scale from 1 to 10. *Source* Eurofound (2017, p. 16)

Dimensions of Well-Being	Bottom group	Top group
Missing social support	**12 % - 15 %**	**1 % - 3 %**
Country Codes	GR, LU, ITA	FI, SL, HU
Feeling very unsafe	**10 % - 15 %**	**1 % - 3%**
Country Codes	GR, HU, BG	FI, SL, PO
Trust in others	**4,2 – 5,2**	**6,5 – 8,3**
Country Codes	FR, CY, BG	FI, SE, DE
Social Justice Index	**3,7 – 4,0**	**7,2 – 7,5**
Country Codes	GR, RO, BG	FI, SE, DE

Fig. 11.2 Precarious dimensions of well-being in EU Member States in 2013 and 2016. *Sources* Missing social support: EU (2015, p. 152) (Not having anyone to rely on in case of need); Feeling very unsafe: EU (2015, p. 167) (Feeling very unsafe when walking alone at night); Trust in others: EU (2015, pp. 197, 207) (measured with eleven-point scale); Social Justice Index: Social Justice: Bertelsmann Stiftung, Index Report 2016; Social Inclusion Monitor

support relations above 80%. Northern countries are in a better position, which is documented in Ireland, Denmark and Sweden with having support ratios of more than 95%. Again a sufficient support culture is more available in Northern Europe, but also in Southern Europe, the perceived missing of the help of friends and relatives is in the average rather low (OECD 2011, p. 174). In EU countries, social support is available in the eyes of the people in a rather sufficient amount. A surprising tendency is that countries with a more developed welfare state are also characterized by stronger network support.

Feelings of unsafety. Safety is basic for quality of life and with respect to physical safety people in Europe see deficits as well as contributions to well-being. A typical situation in European countries, where people tend to develop anxieties is when they are walking alone at night. The results for such kind of question indicate that anxieties during a night walk in the environment are a minor problem. 6.8% say they would feel very unsafe during the night walk compared with 28.4% of people who feel safe. The majority of the inhabitants of the EU feel fairly safe, and another part feels a bit unsafe. A very unsafe feeling exists predominantly in Bulgaria, Greece and Hungary (EU 2015, p. 167). People feel most safe in Slovakia, Finland and the Netherlands.

This again is an example that deficits of quality of life in special dimensions are concentrated on certain countries. In general, security during night walks is no dominant problem. But it can be that new threats recently came up due to terroristic actions, and therefore, the walk at night is no longer the typical threat of people. New threats of safety and the feeling of safety seem to have been developed and can influence the feeling of safety in the future negative.

Trust in others. Trust is a fundamental resource for the functioning of human societies, may it be related to other people, to institutions or to rules. If trust would be missing, we would lose our capability to act efficient and reliable. Trust is with respect to quality of life of high importance because it has irreplaceable functions. When people in Europe are asked if they trust others than the result is in comparison with the usual satisfaction ratings rather low (Ahrendt et al. 2015, p. 649/50).[1] In the year 2013, the average rating of trust in Europe is close to 5.8 on the eleven-point scale (EU 2015, p. 207) and seems low compared with similar measurements. The differences between the countries trust levels are extraordinary high and vary between 4.2 and 8.3.

Trust is high among the people in Denmark, Finland and Sweden on the one side and low in Bulgaria, Cyprus, and France on the other side. Again we see a broad middle field with many countries having trust in others around the EU average of 5.8 Among the trust in institutions, for example, trust into the political system, trust into the legal system, there is the trust into the police to whom trust is the highest in the European Union (EU 2015, p. 207). This positive reputation and the factual behaviour of the police should be kept in balance.

All in all trust is a scarce but important resource in the EU. All societies in the EU are challenged to beware and improve their level of trust. The trust level among people

---

[1] The concept of trust was used at Eurofound some years before the Eurostat survey, but the scales are different and the results are therefore not comparable.

in some countries seems extremely low. Life is more difficult if trust is missing. The countries with a high amount of trust are the same countries, which show the highest satisfaction.

Social Justice. Social justice, as people feel it, is not very well investigated, though it is an important feature of our societies. In various country studies have found, that people are not convinced that their life is just or fair. The concept of social justice—as experts define the problem—has been adapted in a Europe-wide study which shows very different results for the EU member countries. According to the index of "social justice" (Bertelsmann Stiftung 2016), a comprehensive evaluation of social justice for all countries of the European Union was developed.

The Social Justice Index is related to the participation chances of individuals and contains 6 dimensions and 36 indicators. The dimensions are at risk of poverty and social exclusion, educational policy, employment rate, social inclusion policy health policy and family policy. Each country collects points according to their performance which sums up in the best case to 7.51 for Sweden, followed by Finland and Denmark, and in the opposite case to 3.66 for Greece, which is close to Bulgaria and Romania. Four studies are available up to now since 2008.

The outcomes confirm the previously found results from this and other studies: Greece remains often the tail lamp of the comparisons. The distance between Greece on rank 28 to the countries of Romania (rank 27) and Bulgaria (rank 26) has increased recently. The Nordic States, Sweden with Finland and Denmark, were able to keep their top position over time. But according to the measurements from the years 2007/2008, these states had all in all losses with respect to social justice (Bertelsmann Stiftung 2016). It is not wrong to speak of a precarious situation for the development of social justice.

Summary. This data about living arrangements and ways of life give an idea, why well-being in Europe is high but also fragile and precarious. To live alone in a household is an increasing style of life though this living style is accompanied in the past by rather low life satisfaction. An advantage for well-being in Europe is that social support seems to be a rich resource in Europeans everyday life. The feeling of unsafety during a night walk in Europe is not very strong. The impression from trust measurement in Europe seems not very high for trust. There is room for developing more trust in many European countries. Most social deficits exist with respect to justice within the society, and it seems a difficult task to convince people from more justice and fairness in society.

All in all the picture of successful and less successful societies is very clear. Bulgaria and Greece are most often in the bottom area, and Finland is the top land which is in each case on a top position. In Finland people are less missing social support as in other countries, they do not feel anxious during their night walks they have more trust in others and the justice index is highest. Greece people have more anxious feelings, less trust and less justice; Bulgarian people are confronted with less support, less trust and less justice. The member states of the EU are challenged by inequalities and discrepancies which wait for a political answer.

References

Ahrendt, D., Dubois, H., & Mezger, E. (2015). An overview of quality of life and well-being in Europe. In W. Glatzer, L. Camfield, V. Moller, & M. Rojas (Eds.), *Global handbook of quality of life* (p. 640). Dordrecht: Springer.

Bertelsmann Stiftung. (2016). *Social justice in the EU—Index report 2016*. Social Inclusion Monitor Europe.

Eurofound. (2017). *European quality of life survey 2016. Quality of life, quality of public services, and quality of society*. Luxembourg: Publications Office of the European Union.

European Union. (2015). *Quality of life—Facts and views*. Luxembourg: Eurostat, Statistical Books.

OECD. (2011). *How's life. Measuring well-being*. Paris: OECD Publishing.

OECD. (2014). *Society at a Glance 2014. OECD Social Indicators*. Paris: OECD Publishing.

Chapter 12
Long-Term Change and Future Perspectives

Abstract This chapter is a summary chapter and gives a long view back from ancient times up to modernity. Peoples and collective events are changing, and societies were transformed and create new constellations of well-being. With respect to the state of well-being, it does not seem stable and sustainable but, moreover, fragile and precarious. It is difficult to attain a high level of well-being for a society and then to support the different levels of well-being, to keep the high levels, to stabilize and enforce the middle levels and to support and increase well-being at the lower strata.

Long-term change. The historical development of people on the European continent is regarded since five large populations shaped the continent about 3000 years ago: Celts, Greeks, Romans, Germanics and Slavs built early civilizations and laid ground for the improvement of well-being in Europe. The performance of these early civilizations was sustainable, and some of their contributions are available up today. The Celts developed long roads through Europe; the Greeks created a cultural model for other peoples; the Germanics demonstrated how to shelter woods and forests; from the Slavs, we could learn how to grow to the biggest European tribe at the less advantageous regions of Eastern Europe. The lesson from the Romans is now to organize a big empire which strives for the goals of peace, prosperity and satisfaction.

When the Roman Empire broke down social stability in Europe disappeared for some hundred years and a lot of "unrest" did not allow much "well-being". Especially during the Great European Migration, the peoples of Europe were exposed to turbulence. A new distribution of empires and kingdoms emerged, and the societal transformations led finally to the Empire of Charlemagne, which can be regarded as a first European state on European territory. But for the next thousand years, the development went away from Europe's unification. The "Franconian Empire" was dissolved in multiple territories and independent states emerged which were carrying a lot of wars among another. During many wars in Europe's medieval history, millions of peoples were killed and human living conditions were destroyed. Dissatisfaction due to violence affected the people of Europe at many times and in many territories. Additional plagues and famines brought severe pains to the populations in Europe. Finally, the World War I and World War II were destroying broad regions in

Europe and increased the number of fatalities from wars by new technical weapons. Whenever peoples seemed to recover from a disaster often the next one stood before the door. In these times, satisfaction with life never could emerge in the long run in a sustainable way. Nevertheless in these historical times, an improvement of living conditions happened. Health improved and consequently life expectation was prolonged, economic productivity increased and improved the level of material living conditions which concerned wealth, income, consumption and nutrition; political participation was implemented and suffrage was granted, first to men then also to women. The spread of democracy enlarged peoples influence on their governments and enforced peoples claims for their well-being.

But success is only half of the story of history. In each dimension of well-being, counter processes emerged. People in Europe were confronted with new health threats as previously unknown infectious diseases appeared; economic growth reached in the course of time its "limits to growth" and had to take into consideration the negative consequences of uncontrolled growth for environment and climate. The establishment of democracies increased people's influence on their governments, but democracy lost its glory when it was implemented in everyday life. In a mixture of progress and regress, there were tendencies to improve and to deteriorate well-being at the same time.

Main historical steps of development which laid to increasing well-being in Europe were the foundation of nation-states, the breakthrough of industrialization, the spread of democracy and the institutionalization of the welfare state. The whole process of societal development is described with the concepts of civilization and modernization. It has arrived now at the challenges of globalization.

European nations were historically engaged again and again in wars. After the bad experience with the wars in the twentieth century, it came to an increase of the acceptance of international cooperation and supranational unification. The European Union is an extraordinary example, that it is possible to transform a continent of enemy nations into a relatively peaceful relationship of peoples. There is now a successful peacetime after World War II since about 70 years.

Future perspectives. What can people in Europe expect for their future well-being, given the societal tendencies of today? To keep well-being in the future as it is today a first recommendation would be to pay sufficient attention to well-being and not to ignore the threats. Satisfaction with life should be a serious concern of the people, and it is a precious good that is difficult to attain and to sustain on higher levels. Satisfaction with life is no sufficient indicator for the well-being of individuals and societies, but a society without life satisfaction is not worth living.

Critics of the satisfaction concept exist since the ancient Greek philosophers. But they seem to have misunderstood the tricky meaning of satisfaction. As far as we can see, everybody wants satisfaction with the own lifestyle. In special cases can happen that somebody is satisfied with its state of dissatisfaction. The preferences of individuals know different sources of satisfaction. This is a problem for modern democracies that the sources for satisfaction of the people are not homogenous and partly contradictory.

One of the most interesting sources of satisfaction is that satisfaction results from the assistance of other human beings, who are in need or emergency. On the background of social inequality, it is necessary that human beings are equipped with social characteristics as social support, solidarity, helpfulness, compassion and similar attitudes. The result of various studies is, that people, who are more satisfied with their own life spend more time and resources to take care for others. Perhaps this relationship is the rescue of a positive future image of our societies. A society, which provides social cohesion, social inclusion and solidarity for all will attain a higher level of well-being than a society which excludes the disadvantaged and poor ones.

The risk of well-being is that it is fragile and precarious. Fragile means well-being is easily broken and lacking in substance. The tension lines within each society are not sure. The gender balance can break when men do not accept the catch up of women and women take positions of men above the balance. The balance between age groups and generations is still a problem, and intergenerational justice is a topic. Education leads into trouble when more and more well-educated people try to find privileged jobs which are not available. The benefits of higher education will be missing. The balance between rich and poor will not keep when the discrepancy between the low and high levels of the income pyramid will explode. An inequality increase is foreseeable because in the global economy there are nearly unlimited possibilities to accumulate income and wealth in a few hands. Finally the balance between authentic people and migrants will afford that migrants have fair chance. If there are distortions, then this is a danger that well-being breaks.

Well-being is precarious in the sense, i.e. uncertain, insecure and unstable. More and more people are living alone which is no contribution to the well-being of individuals. The accommodations of the households have been attained at high levels in the past, but now it seems that scarcity and expensiveness have created a new problem. The well-being of jobs, which is a typical concern of the labour unions, seems to be threatened more in times of globalization. Education is a master key for creating life satisfaction, but it seems to lose its distributing power. The unequal levels of living will raise the question for what inequality is good. In most European countries, the trust in other people is low and this should be regarded as a warning sign.

Another precariousness is a consequence of the dynamic and often cyclical development of the worlds capitalist economies. After a crisis, which hurts the people, normally a boom arises and brings satisfaction. The rise and decline of nations happen for sure (Olson 1982). The well-being and quality-of-life research profits from the activities of many organizations which are engaged in rescuing the planet Earth like, for example the Club of Rome (Weizsäcker et al. 2018). Hopefully their success will lead to attain a better balance between progress and regress in Europe.

For Europe's future, the well-being developments on its main paths will be decisive. State- and nation-building will go on, not backward to independent nations moreover forward to the stabilization of supranational bonds at the continent. At the same time, regional territories should be enforced and they should receive far-reaching autonomy to build their own living conditions and their quality of life.

The developmental cooperation with the north of Africa and near East should be improved. Economic growth could go on if it is qualitatively controlled. The production of goods and bads should be evaluated carefully from the contribution to human wel -being. Environmental damage should be avoided, and sustainable consumption should be supported. Europe and its states need to improve their democratic content on the different levels of local, regional, national and supranational institutions. People should receive more authentic participation and increase trust in government and collective institutions according to their performance. The welfare state should combine self-sufficiency for most people with efficient social support for the needy ones. The modification of income distribution should be acceptable according to fair burdens and public needs. Europe's march to more well-being in the future is long, but the way behind was much longer (Fig. 12.1).

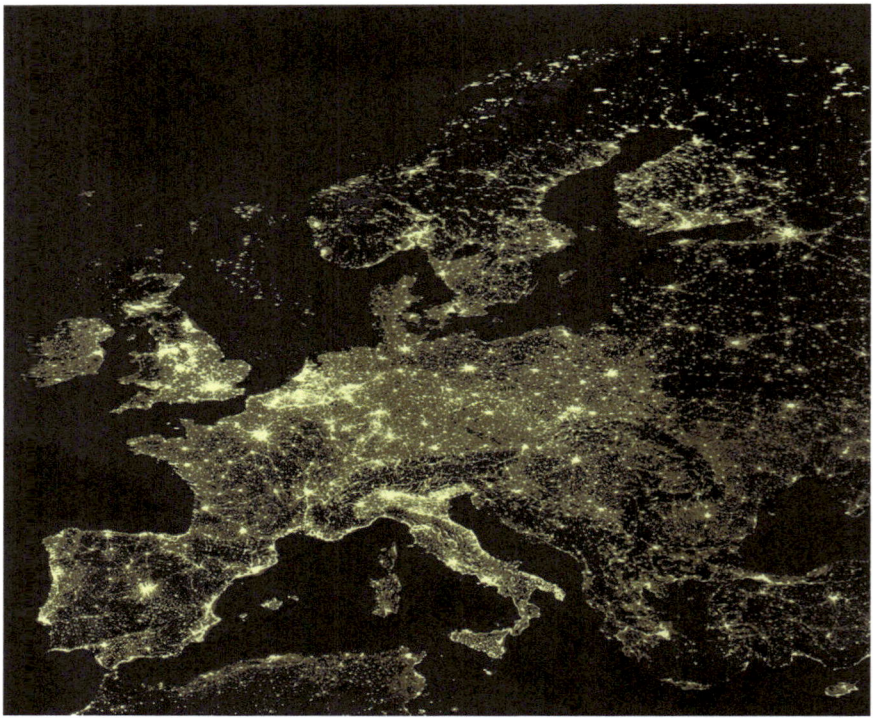

Fig. 12.1 Europe at night from above. *source* https://commons.wikimedia.org/wiki/File%3A Earthlights_2002.jpg

References

Olson, M. (1982). *The rise and decline of nations: Economic growth, Stagflation and Social Rigidities*. New Haven and London: Yale University Press.

Weizsäckerm E. U., & Wijkman, A. (2018). Wir sind dran. Club of Rome: Der große Bericht. Gütersloher Verlagshaus.

Appendix
Methodological Remarks on Social Reporting about Well-Being in Historical and International Context

Abstract There is a widespread need for the long-term historical reconstruction of societal developments. In this study, the history of European's well-being is on the proof. Well-being is a recognized goal since ancient times. In the Roman Empire, people spoke of peace, prosperity and satisfaction these goals were partly transformed but are still alive in modern time. Explicit measurement of well-being developed in the past decades to a task of social sciences and international organizations. Modern data production was institutionalized all over the world and representative survey became a key instrument for the diagnosis of the structural changes of nations, continents and the world. Social indicators and quality-of-life research were combined with an interest in social reporting. Monitoring social change is a recognized instrument which is used to receive knowledge about the societies and their development and to be responsible to the needs of people.

This comprehensive socio-historic and international report concerns well-being developments in Europe. Thanks to the intellectual support from historical personalities, like "Marcus Tullius Cicero" from Rome and "Johann Wolfgang Goethe" from Frankfurt, who are cited at the beginning of the book, the long-term approach adapted in this article received friendly encouragement. Both personalities expressed an extraordinary support for the socio-historical time span of this article regarding 3000 years of human development.

If well-being was always a recognized goal in historical and modern societies is in doubt, clearly there were authoritarian political regimes which ignored the well-being of people. But as it seems most people of modern Europe would prefer for their life "peace, prosperity and satisfaction" if it is adapted to modern conditions. It is the burden of human development that there were always mighty people and groups which brought destruction, sorrow and dissatisfaction over Europe and the world. Well-being has sometimes been a master goal and also often a by-product of societal tendencies, and sometimes, it has been neglected. Well-being in its emphatic sense was never realized. People live always between hopes for well-being and fears that they could lose peace, miss prosperity and diminish satisfaction.

The stimulating idea of postulating quality of life came from welfare theorists (Pigou 1909/1920) and the interest in social indicators for measuring well-being was early shared between social sciences and supranational institutions (Bauer 1965; OECD 1974, 1976). In recent years, the conceptual and practical knowledge about well-being and social reporting were summarized through overviews in the EU context. Social scientists recommend social indicators to the European Union (Atkinson et al. 2001). Measuring progress in a changing world was the topic of a European Commission (Commission of the European Community 2009). The limits of economic measurement and the direction for social progress were content of another European study (Stiglitz et al. 2009) and the proposal about the goal of "Well-being for All" profited especially from the engagement of the Council of Europe (Council of Europe 2008, 2011). Well-being became a central goal of mankind which enriched traditional debates about the pursuit of human well-being and their advances (Estes and Sirgy 2018).

The historical analysis of well-being is confronted with the main problem to find within an endless number of historical events and processes which ones are important and which one can be neglected for the given task. Selective decisions have to be made all the time about the relevance of topics and it is nearly impossible to go into details. There is no chance to explain in a short study for all the 28 EU countries how they attained their special position in Europe. And it would be impossible to look for all the 28 countries which subgroups of their population had some progress for their well-being and which one lost partly their well-being. Readers have to accept that it is not European Commission possible to have both, the broad overview and the detailed exploration. This study is concentrated on events and structures which are most significant for the constitution of well-being in the history of Europe.

A basic decision in well-being and quality-of-life research is to look on social and historical processes from two views: namely, first how people perceive themselves their lives and their society, and second, how is the awareness of social events and social processes from the eyes of other people especially from experts or interested people. What the experts describe is often designed as "objective" and what ordinary people report is called their "subjective" reality. Well-being developments cannot be traced without being perceived and assessed either in the view of experts or in the eyes of the people who participate in the events. Since centuries in many publications, historical or philosophical experts tell how they evaluate from their perspective historical processes and societies. In recent decades, an increasing number of survey studies asked how people see their society and their lives.[1] Knowledge about this topic could be important for supporting cohesion and peace in Europe. Often we find social reports in which objective living conditions are

---

[1]In an early study, an interesting perspective was implemented by the question "how nations see each other" (Buchanan and Cantril 1953).

diagnosed in combination with the subjective perception of the people. Among the critical topics, the problem of inequality within and between European societies attains much attention.

In social reporting, the idea is emphasized to publish not only for scientific experts but also for intelligent readers who are interested in the subject. The intention of social reporting in this study is to present adequate information for European people, who may be interested in their own well-being history, and to people from abroad, who want to be informed about the well-being history of their European neighbours. Of course, the two groups will have more or less pre-knowledge and different expectations, which cannot be met all the time. Complex methodological approaches and elaborations, which are difficult to follow, are here avoided. Social reporting emphasizes the point that people who are subject of social research should be able to understand the research results.

A further problem of this type of socio-historical and international comparable study is the data which are available for describing the socio-historical and international processes (Sirgy et al. 2017). Most often we find in the quality-of-life literature single country or population group studies which came up early and went ahead of comparative studies. One of the first studies in Europe on quality of life and well-being was published in 1984 under the title "Lebensqualität in Deutschland" (Glatzer and Zapf 1984). From the preference for structural information stems the support for representative survey data. Only with the help of representative data, a complex and differentiated unit as Europe can be characterized without getting lost in details. For modern times, it is no problem to find structural data because data production has attained a high level.

Most important structural, historical and international comparable data for the EU are produced and collected at the following statistical and data units.

Overview of Country Indicators for the 28 EU Member States and the most World Countries

European Union/Eurofound (2017). European Quality of Life Survey, 2016. Nearly 37,000 interviews with 1000–2000 per country in 28 European member states and 5 EU-candidates. Carried through earlier in 2003, 2007 and 2011.

European Union/Eurostat (2015). Quality of Life—Facts and Views. The European statistical agency with its first quality of life survey in 2015. Includes EU with 28 countries and some additional ones.

European Union/Eurostat (2015). Quality of Life—Facts and Views. The European statistical agency with its first quality of life survey in 2015. Includes EU with 28 countries and some additional ones.

OECD (2014). Van Zanden et al. (eds.) (2014). How Was Life? Global Wellbeing Since 1820. OECD Publishing. "Trends are charted for 25 countries, 8 world regions and the world economy as a whole." This Report gives a summary of own and official data sources.

(continued)

(continued)

OECD (2016). Society at a Glance. OECD Social Indicators. Overview of Social Trends in 35 OECD-Countries and selected Partner Countries.
OECD (2017). How's Life 2017? Measuring well-being. OEC. D Publishing. This is a statistical report, released every two years, that describes some of the essential aspects of life that shape people's well-being in OECD and partner countries.
United Nations (2016). Human Development Report—Human Development for Everyone (2016). Includes the Human Development Index (HDI), which is defined as a welfare measure of the United Nations including the components of health, education and level of living since 1990. It is available for most countries of the world.
World Happiness Report (2018). ed. by Helliwell J, Layard R & Sachs J (2018). The survey 2017 is concerned with global happiness and includes 156 countries (containing the EU-countries) in respect to their happiness levels and 117 countries by the happiness levels of their immigrants. World Happiness reports are available since 2012.
World Database of Happiness (Veenhoven 1995). Research findings on subjective enjoyment of life for most countries of the world including Europe. This data archive is a collection of all quality of life related survey data.

European Union/Eurofound (2017). European Quality of Life Survey, 2016. Nearly 37,000 interviews with 1000–2000 per country in 28 European member states and 5 EU-candidates. Carried through earlier in 2003, 2007 and 2011.

European Union/Eurostat (2015). Quality of Life—Facts and Views. The European statistical agency with its first quality of life survey in 2015. Includes EU with 28 countries and some additional ones.

OECD (2014). Van Zanden et al. (eds.) (2014). How Was Life? Global Wellbeing Since 1820. OECD Publishing. "Trends are charted for 25 countries, 8 world regions and the world economy as a whole." This Report gives a summary of own and official data sources.

OECD (2016). Society at a Glance. OECD Social Indicators. Overview of Social Trends in 35 OECD-Countries and selected Partner Countries.

OECD (2017). How's Life 2017? Measuring well-being. OEC. D Publishing. This is a statistical report, released every two years, that describes some of the essential aspects of life that shape people's well-being in OECD and partner countries.

United Nations (2016). Human Development Report—Human Development for Everyone (2016). Includes the Human Development Index (HDI), which is defined as a welfare measure of the United Nations including the components of health, education and level of living since 1990. It is available for most countries of the world.

---

[2]In the quality-of-life literature, different scales are used from three steps to one hundred steps, which makes comparisons sometimes impossible. In this summary, mostly scales from 0 to 10 and 1 to 10 are in use.

World Happiness Report (2018). ed. by Helliwell J, Layard R & Sachs J (2018). The survey 2017 is concerned with global happiness and includes 156 countries (containing the EU-countries) in respect to their happiness levels and 117 countries by the happiness levels of their immigrants. World Happiness reports are available since 2012.

World Database of Happiness (Veenhoven 1995). Research findings on subjective enjoyment of life for most countries of the world including Europe. This data archive is a collection of all quality of life related survey data.

In most of these data sources, a new scale-type is adapted, which was not in use some decades ago. A main construct is directed towards satisfaction, towards satisfaction with life and towards satisfaction in different life domains. It was measured most often with a scale running from 0 to 10,[2] which means from "not at all satisfied" to "fully satisfied". This scale was used in hundreds of surveys and well-being researcher trust in the measurement method. It is helpful to remember some of the various scales which are broadly accepted, e.g., the medical pain scale (from 0 to 10), the Parker wine scale (from 50 to 100), the Beaufort wind strength scale (from 0 to 12) or the earthquake Richter magnitude scale from (1 to 9). Many people are adapted to this style of thinking and they know that value on a scale is high and what is low. For the interpretation of satisfaction scales, it is recommended to give attention to the results of the many available studies. Values of 9 and 10 are extremely seldom. Values below the scale middle point of "5" are extremely low scores and they are results only in few cases. Small changes in the average on the satisfaction ladder indicate big steps in reality.

It is of general interest to monitor social change and some studies do this explicitly and repeat their surveys in short or long distance. For a profound analysis of recent change of well-being in Europe, it would be necessary to compare all available surveys and to proof, if the changes in time are consistent. Most supranational studies have a small section what is going on in recent times. For a deeper understanding, one should know what groups in the society were the agents of change. The satisfaction with the living standard could increase for the higher strata or for the lower-income strata, which makes a lot of difference for society. Also, it is important if an increase of well-being is a short-term result or a longer-trend phenomenon, which is stable over time. In general, well-being should be monitored how it is attained, sustained and improved over many years. Everybody should be aware that it is a difficult task to identify, to protect and to reproduce well-being in the course of times.

---

[2] In the quality-of-life literature, different scales are used from three steps to one hundred steps, which makes comparisons sometimes impossible. In this summary, mostly scales from 0 to 10 and 1 to 10 are in use.

References

Atkinson, T., Cantillon, B., Marlier, E., & Nolan, B. (2001). *The EU and social indicators*. Oxford: Oxford University Press.

Buchanan, W., & Cantril, H. (1953). *How Nations see each other*. Westport, Connecticut: Greenwood Press Publishers.

Council of Europe. (2008). *Well-being for all. Concepts and tools for social cohesion*. Strasbourg: Council of Europe Publishing.

Commission of the European Community. (2009). *GDP and beyond. Measuring progress in a changing World*. Brussels: COM.

Eurostat. (2015). *Quality of life—Facts and views. Statistical books*. Luxembourg: Publications office of the European Union.

Eurofound. (2017). *European quality of life survey 2016. Quality of life, quality of public services and quality of society*. Luxembourg: Publication Office of the European Union.

Estes, R., & Sirgy, J. (2017). *The Pursuit of human well-being*. Switzerland: Springer International Publishing.

Glatzer, W., & Zapf, W. (1984). Lebensqualität in der Bundesrepublik. Frankfurt: Campus.

Glatzer, W., & Kohl, J. (2017). The History of Well-being in Europe. In R. Estes & J. Sirgy (Eds.), *The Pursuit of human well-being*. Switzerland: Springer International Publishing.

Hellwell, J. F., Layard, H., & Sachs J. D. (2018). World Happiness Report 2018.

Michalos, A. (2014). *Encyclopedia of Well-being and quality of life research*. Dordrecht: Springer.

OECD. (2016). *Society at a glance. OECD social indicators*.

OECD. (2017). *How's life? Measuring well-being*. OECD Publishing.

Olson, M. (1985). *The rise and decline of nations. Economic growth, stagflation and social rigidities*. New Haven and London: Yale University Press.

Pigou, C. E. (1920/2009). *Welfare economics*. New Brunswick, New Jersey: Transaction Publisher

Sirgy, M. J., Estes, R. J., & Selian, A. N. (2017). How we measure well-being: The data: Behind the history of well-being. In R. Estes & J. Sirgy (Eds.), *The pursuit of human well-being*. Switzerland: Springer International Publishing.

Stiglitz, J., Sen, A., & Fitoussi, J. P. (2009). *Report of the commission on the measurement of economic performance and social progress*. www-stiglitz-sen-fitoussi.fr

United Nations. (2016). *Human development report—human development for everyone*. UNDP: hdr.undp.org/en/2016.report

Van Zanden, J. L. (2014). *How was life? Global well-being since 1820*. Luxembourg: OECD Publishing.

Veenhoven, R. (1995). World database of happiness. In *Social indicators research* (Nr. 34 Vol. 3, pp. 299–313).

Weizsäckerm E. U., & Wijkman, A. (2018). Wir sind dran. Club of Rome: Der große Bericht. Gütersloher Verlagshaus.